D0114584

SEX LIVES OF WIVES

SEX LIVES OF WIVES

REIGNITING THE PASSION

HOLLY H. HOLLENBECK

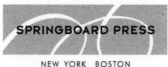

SPRINGBOARD PRESS

NEW YORK   BOSTON

Springboard Press

Hachette Book Group USA
1271 Avenue of the Americas, New York, NY 10020
Visit our Web site at www.HachetteBookGroupUSA.com

First Edition: September 2006

Important Notice:
All cases and characters in this book are composites of acquaintances and Web site
survey participants. Names and details have been changed to ensure privacy and
confidentiality.

　　　This book is not intended as a substitute for advice from trained professionals,
counselors, therapists, doctors, or other mental health professionals. Check with your
mental health provider before altering your therapeutic regimen.

The Ted Kooser quote on page vii is from *Local Wonders: Seasons in the Bohemian Alps*,
University of Nebraska Press, 2002.

Library of Congress Cataloging-in-Publication Data

Hollenbeck, Holly H.
　　Sex lives of wives : reigniting the passion / by Holly H. Hollenbeck — 1st ed.
　　　p. cm.
　　ISBN-10: 0-8212-5808-7 (hardcover)
　　ISBN-13: 978-0-8212-5808-8 (hardcover)
　　1. Married women — Sexual behavior. 2. Wives — Sexual behavior. 3. Sex in
marriage. I. Title.

　　HQ29.H65 2006
　　646.7'8 — dc22   2005033284

10　9　8　7　6　5　4　3　2　1

Q-FF

Book design by Meryl Sussman Levavi
Printed in the United States of America

THIS BOOK IS DEDICATED TO
PASSION SEEKERS EVERYWHERE

And to my mother,
from whom I inherited the passion within

And to my husband, with whom I seek the passion

If you can awaken
inside the familiar
and discover it new,
you need never
leave home.

— TED KOOSER
U.S. poet laureate and
Pulitzer Prize winner

CONTENTS

ACKNOWLEDGMENTS

First and foremost I acknowledge and thank my dear husband, with whom I continue a never-ending quest for passion, knowing so much more of the best is yet to come. Thank you for your love and devotion.

I greatly thank my dear girlfriends for their friendship, humor, support, and encouragement. They are my passion quest support group. Their comments and insights turned a journal of collected stories into an inspirational book and brought about the birth of the Passion Seekers. I especially thank my dear friend Stephanie Murphy and my mother, Helen Marie Nolen. Their encouraging suggestions, insights, and devoted support made all the difference in the writing process. Equally important are all the women and men who shared with me the personal, intimate details of their journeys seeking passion. Their heartfelt, emotion-filled trials and tribulations have helped us find our own way on the passion journey with our long-term mate. Their stories are our compass and map through the pitfalls, detours, and roadblocks along the way.

I thank and greatly acknowledge author Peter Greenberg for his sound advice. If it were not for that chance meeting in the Chicago airport in the summer of 2004, I may never have been inspired to publish all the stories of passion I had uncovered. I also thank author Susan Page, whose book *The Shortest Distance Between You and a Published Book* provided all I needed to know and whose own relationship advice has helped so many. Her encouragement has been invaluable.

I am very thankful for the experience and patience of two incredible professionals: my agent, Joelle Delbourgo, and my editor, Karen Murgolo, whose wisdom, professionalism, and insight have been a blessing. I also greatly thank my publisher, Jill Cohen, for her enthusiasm and exceptionally clear vision for my book as part of the new imprint Springboard Press. Thank you also to copyeditor Karen Landry for all her hard work. Her thoroughness was immensely appreciated. And I thank all the fantastic people at Springboard Press / Hachette Book Group USA, especially my publicist, Matthew Ballast, for his undying commitment to spreading the Passion Seeker enthusiasm.

Thank you to Passion Seekers everywhere. May your continual journeys be blessed with many intimate, passion-filled moments of pleasure and joy.

AUTHOR'S NOTE

People have asked me why I decided to write this book and reveal so much about the sex lives of wives. The answer is simple: there are millions and millions of women (and men) in long-term relationships who *miss the passion* of those early days and wonder what else to try. Some have just plain lost touch with the joy and intimacy that comes with having sexual passion in their lives. According to the U.S. Census Bureau, around 50 percent of first marriages in the United States end in divorce, and additional studies (detailed in chapter 1) reveal that a great many couples are experiencing infidelity issues. An alarming number of married people are now admitting to frequent cybersex and even to having affairs and unconventional sex, and this number is also on the rise (see "The Current Estimates for the United

States" in chapter 1). I wanted to know why so many people were venturing down these paths *and* how these choices were affecting their relationships at home. I wanted to know how to protect my own relationship and how to ensure that my husband and I were doing everything we could, and everything we should, to keep the passion alive.

I searched for answers in many self-help books written by therapists, doctors, and sex experts. I read about the 101 ways to "do it" better. I started asking anyone who would talk to me what their secrets were and what they had learned from their own trials and tribulations. I organized the first passion quest support group, which evolved into the Passion Seekers' Club. I started my Web site survey and an online exchange of ideas, and I conducted hundreds of interviews. The stories I accumulated fascinated me and inspired me to put more effort and energy into my own relationship. When I discussed all of this with my friends, I discovered that the support and knowledge we could share with one another were enlightening and motivating. But even more important than that, I realized that just a little bit of focus on our sexual self could make a dramatic difference in our marriage, and *not* just in the bedroom.

There has been a lot that I have learned from my research into the real-life journeys of others who are seeking the passion. One of the most important pieces of wisdom that I have gleaned from my research is this: relationships require an element of optimism — a hope for the future and a belief that more of the best is yet to come. We hear and make enough negative comments about our relationships. Instead, we need to be encouraged and inspired to continually seek passion with our mate. Thus, I selected stories for this book that not only taught some important lessons but also revealed, through the successes and failures of others, how to rediscover the passion and how perhaps not to.

Please note that this book sets out in detail the actual experiences of the many people I have met and interviewed, visitors to my Web site, and Internet chat buddies. All the stories are true, with the identifying information altered to protect those who took a risk by sharing their experiences with me.

There is nothing scientific here — just real-life efforts by real-life people to keep the passion alive. We can buy all the latest sex-technique books telling us how to "do it" better, but these will not likely reveal what people are really doing and what is really working, or not working, *and* why. This book explores reality and provides sexy, intimate stories of the tried-and-true, and also includes Passion Seekers' tips that can really work to bring fun and fantasy back into our lives. *Sex Lives of Wives* reveals paths to avoid and paths that lead us to — and not away from — our ultimate goal: an intimate and passionate *long-term* relationship. Let the sex begin!

HOLLY H. HOLLENBECK
Founder of PassionSeekers.com

SEX LIVES
OF WIVES

INTRODUCTION

MISSING THE PASSION — THE WOMEN ARE TALKING

For effect, she moaned and stroked his chest. Her husband was on top of her, doing his thing, but she was not really there. She was wondering if she remembered to throw the wash into the dryer and if she forgot to turn the television off in the family room. It was not always like this for her, but often enough it was. She tried to focus her mind on the sensation, but tonight it was no use. Tonight it was just another chore before turning over and finally getting some sleep.

Whether having cocktails with my friends, working out in the gym, attending scrapbooking parties, getting together with others during the lunch hour, or browsing Web site chat rooms, I am constantly hearing the same comments from women in committed relationships: "What sex life?" "Well, since the kids . . ."

"He is constantly complaining about our sex life." "The passion is gone from our relationship." These statements are so common that I am actually shocked when I hear a positive comment from a married person about his or her sex life. I asked close friends about the passion in their relationship (or the lack thereof). I followed discussions and read articles on the Internet and even started a poll on my Web site. I would ask: Why do so many couples in long-term relationships have virtually nonexistent sex lives with their mates or minimally satisfying ones at best?

It is not shocking that so many attitudes about married sex (or even sex in any long-term committed relationship) are predominately *negative*. What is surprising is the number of women who are looking for *and* finding passionate outlets *outside* their committed relationship, either through cybersex or through actual affairs. These women, even with their hectic work schedules and home responsibilities, are finding the time and energy to sneak around and cover their tracks to make room for passionate encounters outside the home. Why are so many women doing this?

Others who are not actually cheating by definition are finding many creative ways to add a thrill or spark of passion to their sex life. They are attending "sexy" nightclubs, showing up at "lifestyle" resorts and events, inviting guests to share their marital beds, and participating in other such activities. As we get older, we read and learn more about people's nonconventional attempts to spice up the sex in their long-term relationship. Are these dramatic efforts successful in heating things up at home?

I have always thought of myself as an extremely passionate person, yet these issues were swirling around in my head as I did an inventory of my own long-term sexual relationship with my husband. What were we doing to keep the passion alive? Was it enough? Was there more that we could try? As women often do, I turned to my girlfriends for their advice and input.

When my friends and I get together, we usually talk (or complain) about the kids, our husbands, our jobs, or the many responsibilities we have. Our group has worn every hat imaginable, from career woman with no children to stay-at-home mom with a plethora of community volunteer commitments. Many of us have taken on several roles, juggling quite a few at the same time. Since I graduated from law school in my early twenties, I have done trial work as a law-firm associate, acted as in-house counsel in the technology industry, performed as a stay-at-home mom, worked part-time over the Internet, volunteered for more charitable projects than I can remember, played the role of executive's wife, and nursed my ill father as he lost his battle with cancer, all the while caring for two children, with their many activities, projects, needs, and interests. Most of us have a long list like this one, and it is exhausting when we think about all that we do and all the roles that we play. Often forgotten from our priorities is the role of sexual and intimate partner in a committed relationship.

A woman's role as a long-term *sexual* partner often gets lost in the shuffle. Sometimes our needs are filled elsewhere. Sometimes we even forget the need, forget we are sexual beings. Thoughts of kids, dishes, laundry, mail, homework, exercising, car pools, errands, volunteer commitments, etc., are dancing through our heads as we lie down at night. We get so busy with the everyday rushing around that often all we wish for by the end of the day is to close our eyes and go to sleep so that we can get up the next day and get "everything" done.

Gone are the early days of our relationship, when we waited in bed in sexy lingerie for our partner to come home. Gone are the days when we did not even make it to the bedroom before we ripped off the other's clothes. Gone are the days of long, leisurely kissing and petting. Gone is the passionate newness of those "honeymoon" days. Do we even have time to notice what is gone? For some of us, the answer is a resounding "Yes," and we have been struggling with what to do about it.

One evening, some of my friends and I were having our regular monthly cocktail "meeting." After trying the newest version of the death-by-chocolate martini (and several of them, I might add), we started talking about our sex lives. We shared the details . . . the good, the bad, and the ugly. We whispered juicy tidbits. We admitted "shameful secrets." We sought one another's counsel in dealing with our "oversexed, demanding" husbands. We laughed and laughed. We had a great time. Later that night, when we got home, every one of our partners got laid. From then on, I referred to our group as the "passion quest support group." This was the birth of the Passion Seekers' Club.

We decided that we *all* needed a little more passion in our lives, a little more "that feels great!" We decided we needed some focus on our often forgotten sexual selves. We talked about what we used to do in the bedroom, what we missed doing, and what was different now. We shared our boredom and our varied attempts to overcome it. We discovered that the key ingredient was our attitude. Somewhere along the line, our attitude about sex changed somewhat. Somewhere amid raising kids and managing a household, attending appointments and keeping up with the work schedules, our intimate sexual relationship with our mate moved way down the list, and all our priorities shifted.

My friends and I made a pact. We decided we would figure this out. We would find the answer to what happened to our

youthful passion for sex with our spouse. We would try something different, something creative, and report back with the
results. Not surprisingly, the efforts we started putting into our
sexual relationships were well received by our mates. So the
challenge continued, and soon we were sharing some juicy
details and feeling more in tune with our sexual selves again.
Although the paths we took were different, each of us was
reporting renewed passion in her intimate relationship.

Intrigued, I sought out the opinions of other couples who
spoke highly of their committed sexual relationships. For those
who were not "newlyweds," I wondered what they were doing
differently. What was their secret? It is astonishing how many
details and amazing stories we will hear if we just ask — whether
in the anonymous atmosphere of a vacation resort, over drinks at
a club, in a chat room on the Internet, or through Web site surveys. As a result of my research, I discovered many creative
approaches to keeping the passion alive.

Soon the research took on a life of its own, and before I realized it, I had uncovered hundreds of positive — and not so positive — experiences to report on. From the stories of the many
people, friends or otherwise, who were willing to talk to me, and
from the opinions I received from reportedly sexually happy
couples, I was able to make some beneficial observations about
how to maintain a passionate sex life in a long-term relationship
and how not to.

This book will explore some of the endless possibilities of
how to reinvent sexual passion in our life and thereby create a
more fulfilling intimate relationship at home. The fascinating
stories I uncovered include pitfalls some have encountered along
the way and how relationships can "weather" them. And we will
see how women just like us have found the inspiration to spice

up their sex life before it is too late. Learning of these experiences will help us to better utilize our instinct, our attitude, and our creativity to produce renewed and continued desire and satisfaction in the bedroom, and ultimately the "feel great" intimacy we crave in our long-term relationship.

CHAPTER ONE

PASSION QUESTS

JOURNEYS BEGIN TO REDISCOVER THE PASSION

WHY SEEK THE PASSION?

Has sex become a chore at home, just another task to complete before we go to sleep? We get so busy taking care of others — our kids, clients, bosses, friends, extended family, etc. — that at times we forget to take care of ourselves and our mate. Sometimes we do not exercise or eat right, let alone make sure we have a healthy dose of sexual interaction. We often are so busy with everything that our sexuality takes a backseat.

Do our sexual needs ever really go away? We are sometimes reminded of those urges when we read a romance novel, when that young trainer leans over to give us a spot in the gym, when the sexy grocery-store clerk smiles at us, or maybe when our coworker flirts with us. We fantasize and masturbate. We remember and imagine. We would like to have the ultimate fantasy: a passionate and intimate relationship — the happily ever after. Why then do we seem to have so little energy to put into our sex life with our mate?

We hear a lot about married women and lost libido. Books are dedicated to the subject of boosting the libido and finding the medical and emotional causes of loss of interest in sex. Of course, there are many situations in which a woman's sex drive is low or nonexistent due to actual physical or emotional problems. These issues and their possible treatments are outside the scope of this book. The issue for many of us, however, is not lost libido but rather our own lack of focus on our sexual needs, or perhaps the misdirection of that focus. We rarely put much time or energy into our sexual relationship with our mate. We need to think about all the effort we devote to our children, our careers, and/or our communities, and then look at how much time we actually give to our sexual relationship. Often there is no comparison. Our sexual relationship is way, way down the list of priorities.

> The issue is our own lack of focus on our sexual needs, or perhaps the misdirection of that focus.

Giving our sexual relationship such a low priority is really hurting us, much more than we care to admit. We are hurt because the intimacy we crave with our mate is lost. We are hurt because our innate sexual needs are being ignored. We are hurt because we are missing out on a lot of "that feels great" in our lives. We can work ourselves like machines, taking care of everyone and everything until we drop at night, then getting up and doing it again the next day. Or we can start paying a little attention to those inner desires again and start feeding them. The rewards will be huge. Those days of looking forward to intimate time alone with our mate will return, and sex will no longer be a chore. Our relationship can only improve when we start putting a little time and effort into seeking passionate encounters.

If we continue to place a low priority on sex, we are only hurting ourselves, and, in the long run, our neglect will have a detrimental effect on even the best of relationships. How does placing a low priority on our sex lives affect our husband or long-term mate? We all know how much the men in our lives value sex, and we need to realize that they value it for many of the same reasons we should value it — the intimacy and closeness it creates with our mate, not to mention the sheer pleasure.

The Seven Reasons to Seek Passion with Our Mate
(Advantages to Placing a High Priority on Our Sexual Relationship)

- Increases intimacy
- Feeds our innate sexual needs
- Provides a lot of "that feels great" in our life
- Improves the overall health of our relationship
- Reduces the risk of becoming a statistic
- Provides a great tension reliever and mood elevator
- Provides a creative outlet and an avenue of great fun

When my friends and I got home from our first unofficial passion quest support meeting, every one of our mates got laid. Having spent some time confiding in our friends about sex, having shared some secrets, having made suggestions, we were suddenly energized to not only have sex but have it *enthusiastically.* Just that little bit of focus on our sex lives triggered the innate desire within us.

Right away, when we began exploring the paths to rediscover the passion, our relationships were dramatically affected — and I am not just talking about in the bedroom. This is because our sexual lives have a powerful and profound effect on our relationships as a whole. The depth of this impact will become crystal clear when we explore the real-life experiences of women who journeyed out, seeking to rediscover their sexual selves and the "passion pot of gold."

One friend of mine told me about the dramatic change in her relationship with her mate when she simply eliminated thirty minutes of nighttime television and instead spent the time "messing around" with him in bed. She decided that she could accomplish a more complete state of relaxation by cuddling and sharing massages with him than she could by passively watching TV. The time together often led to sex, and even when it did not, the small effort on her part did not go unnoticed. Soon her husband was much more agreeable and much more attentive to her needs both in the bedroom and out.

I have made an impact on my own relationship with an effort as small as occasionally buying the latest book on sexual technique and trying something new every time I have sex. This usually results in my husband picking up the book, reading it, and sharing in the application of the "new" sexual approach. (Trust me, putting a book about sex on the nightstand all but guarantees our man will pick it up and look at it.) Some techniques or positions, because of their absurdness, result in fits of laughter, and others my husband and I agree we shall certainly use again. In any case, just that little bit of effort on my part results in a wonderful return in intimacy.

The purpose here is to share real-life sexual experiences — both minor and major — with the goal of helping us find renewed sexual passion in our life. Sometimes the path toward rediscovery is a long and difficult one. Sometimes minor efforts are not enough, and sometimes dramatic efforts have a major negative impact on our relationship. The journeys each of us take to reignite the passion are unique, but the resulting discoveries allow for some universal observations. By sharing experiences with each other, we learn what might work for our relationship and what might not. Learning about each other's mistakes along the way may help us avoid pitfalls and seek more productive paths. Ultimately, we will realize the *need* and the benefit to *actively* seeking a more fulfilling and passionate sex life in our long-term relationship.

AVOID BECOMING A STATISTIC

When I first approached women about their experiences with sex in their long-term relationships, many insisted that all they could contribute was "everything you would want to know about missionary style." And, as an aside, they jokingly offered to share all their "secrets" about how to "get [sex] over with as soon as possible." With this kind of frequent commentary from women in long-term committed relationships, I am not at all surprised by the number of people who are unhappy about their sex lives or, for that matter, having affairs and getting divorced.

My Passion Seeker friends and I conducted an unofficial count of all the women we knew who had an affair or were having an affair. We were shocked by the fact that *each* of us could think of at least two different women, and many of those women were now divorced or living with a strained relationship at home. Granted, some of these women had an affair in retaliation for their spouse's indiscretions, but they were nevertheless cheating (or had cheated) on their mate.

According to the National Opinion Research Center's Reports on Sexual Behavior, the number of wives cheating on their husbands in the United States is on the rise. Their findings show that in the last twelve to fifteen years, the percentage of previously or currently married women who have ever been involved in an extramarital affair has risen while the rate for men has remained about the same. This means that the "infidelity gap" has narrowed. (See "The Current Estimates for the United States" below.) An Internet search will bring up many Web sites geared toward women who are cheating — or wanting to cheat — or men who are looking for married women to cheat with. Reports vary widely as to the actual percentage of women in committed relationships who are cheating in the United States, but some experts put the number as high as 55 percent (see "The Current Estimates for the United States" below).

Letting the passion slip away from our relationship sounds like a quick way to become another statistic — one of the approximately 50 percent divorcing or the estimated 40 to 55 percent having affairs (see the list below). Of course, there are many other stresses on a marriage, but just as most marriage counselors will tell us, discontent in the bedroom is one of the biggest. What are we accomplishing by sticking our head in the sand and trying not to think about how much we miss the passionate newness of those early days?

The Current Estimates for the United States

(See the resources section at the back of this book for a comprehensive list of studies and additional citation detail.)

- About 50 percent of first marriages end in divorce. (U.S. Census Bureau Current Population Reports, February 2002)

- Forty-three percent of first marriages break up within the first fifteen years. (Centers for Disease Control, National Center for Health Statistics, May 2001)

- Tom W. Smith, author of the National Opinion Research Center's Reports on Sexual Behavior (April 2003), notes that "In the last twelve to fifteen years, the 'infidelity gap' has narrowed, as the percent of previously or currently married women ever involved in an affair has risen while the percent of previously or currently married men ever involved in an affair has remained stable."

- Forty-five to 55 percent of married women and 50 to 60 percent of married men engage in extramarital sex at some time during their marriage. (Joan D. Atwood and Limor Schwartz, "Cybersex: The New Affair Treatment Considerations," *Journal of Couple and Relationship Therapy,* vol. 1, #3, 2002)

- Approximately half of all married persons have at least one affair during the course of the relationship. (Mary Stuart, coauthor of *The Divorce Recovery Journal,* 1999)

- Sixty percent of men and 40 percent of women will have an extramarital affair at some point. (Peggy Vaughan, therapist and author of *The Monogamy Myth,* 2003)

- According to an online survey of 38,000 Internet users, respondents devote three hours each week to online sexual exploits, and one in ten respondents said they are addicted to sex and the Internet. (Survey by MSNBC.com and Dr. Alvin Cooper, director of the San Jose Marital Services and Sexuality Center in California; as printed on usatoday.com, Newsbytes News Network, 2001)

Maybe we are already one of these statistics. Maybe we had an affair or cybersex, and maybe we got away with it, but did it help at home? Has the passion improved? Or maybe we have just thought about having an affair. Maybe we are dancing on the edge of infidelity because it makes us feel sexy and desired again. Is whetting our appetite outside the home helping to spice things up with our mate or is it just muddying the waters?

When we think about it, many of us are already seeking passion. Sometimes we just complain about the problem, and sometimes we venture out, actively making poor choices to solve it. Do we even realize that we are already on the journey? Have we actually acknowledged to ourselves that we miss the sexual passion in our relationship? Maybe our instinct, our innate sexuality, is calling out to us to do something about it before it is too late. We may not be listening because of the kids and the job and the chores and what have you. We may not think there is anything that can be done about it. We may believe it is too late, takes too much effort, or is "just the way it is" in a long-term relationship. The passion slips away — end of story.

Well that is *not* the end of the story. We need to pay attention to that voice inside us, the one that is calling out to add some excitement, to find the passion, to add more "that feels great!" We need to take action, follow the path, and begin the journey toward a passionate renewal in our lives. This, in fact, is what many women are doing, some in healthy ways and some in not so healthy ways.

The Six Passion Quest Dead Ends

(Dead Ends to Seeking the Missing Passion in Our Relationship)

- Passively letting the passion continue to slip away
- Believing that this is "just the way it is" in a long-term relationship
- Believing that it is too late to do something about the problem

- Believing we do not have the time or energy to do something about it
- Pursuing sexual passion behind our mate's back (i.e., cheating)
- Failing to recognize (and learn from) the dead-end paths we have already ventured down (e.g., ignoring the problem, or committing adultery or dancing on the edge of it)

DO WE NEED TO BEGIN A "PASSION QUEST" OR ARE WE ALREADY ON ONE?

After much complaining and crying into our beers about our sex lives, my friends and I decided we all needed a little kick in the butt, something to once again motivate us to really put some effort into making love. We would each try something new — something different — and then share the results. We would put our collective minds together to find a solution to the boredom that had become our long-term relationships. We would follow the path that was calling out to us. We would start our journey to rediscover the passion.

As we started off and began to share really personal tidbits with one another, I learned that many women were already "treating" the malaise that was their sex life at home. The "treatments" in some cases were questionable and often made the problem worse. Some were very creative, some involved ignoring the problem, and some were, well, unconventional. Each one of us was on a different journey, but all were seeking the same sexual "pot of gold." We were hoping that we could rediscover that passion we had with our mate in those early heated encounters, that somehow we could re-create the excitement. We hoped that our journey would bring us to that place of many intimate moments of "that feels great" pleasure and joy.

Through the diapers and the night feedings, through the car trips with screaming children and the teenagers missing curfew, through it all, we have often had our sexual selves closeted, struggling to again be realized. Once I started questioning anyone who would talk about their sex life, intimate details began to surface. My research uncovered some intriguing and inspiring real-life dramas. Jessie, for instance, regularly reads romance novels, flirts with her trainer, and now desperately wishes to understand what the big deal is about sex. Nora is facing a soon-to-be-empty nest and a passionless marriage. Courtney, on the other hand, has been "experimenting" a lot. Lisa and her husband have tried nude beaches and are even considering a "wild exploration" (see glossary at the back of this book). And Carla thinks she wants to have an affair, flirts regularly with the men at work, and has frequent cybersex.

When we discussed these women and their stories at our Passion Seekers' meetings, we started putting the focus back onto our sexual selves. We realized that, like these women, our sex drives never really vanished — we were just not paying close attention to the fact that we were already on a journey of sorts. We were all, in our own ways, seeking passion in our lives. We all wanted to be "Passion Seekers."

The passion within us is not dead; it is sometimes dormant or hiding, but it is there, struggling to come out and be fully utilized again, or in some cases for the first time. We want to feel sexy and be noticed again, now that we are mature enough to handle it and know what to do with it (and, boy, do we). We have had children, careers, and many experiences. Most women over thirty-five (and especially those who have had children) will tell you that they are more orgasmic now than ever before. We are at our sexual prime.

The paths we take toward rediscovery are not always smooth ones; bumps and wrong turns are often inevitable. We hope to find the passion within ourselves and within our mate, but often we look the wrong way. We start down a path that heads somewhere else. Sometimes the path leads us to a pitfall and the end of our relationship, but sometimes it leads to exciting discoveries with our lifelong mate and takes us to new unexplored heights.

CONSIDERING THE JOURNEYS OF OTHERS — MEET COURTNEY, NORA, JESSIE, CARLA, AND LISA

We learn a lot from our friends. The successes and failures of others can speak volumes. So I sought out the details of those who have already undertaken journeys to find the lost passion. Hearing the revelations of these women, I discovered the extent of the complications involved with exploration. Just where are our journeys taking us and what can we learn from the journeys of others?

Courtney is currently a stay-at-home mother of three. She is organized to a fault and is constantly planning something. She and her husband of nine years have experimented in the past. They are practically the poster couple for location sex, having tried just about all the imaginable spots to "do it." You would never know this by looking at them. They are the picture-perfect conservative WASP family. They work hard to keep their sex life interesting. The problem now is, what should they try next? How do they crank it up a notch?

Nora has been married for about twenty years and has two

children — one already off to college and one who just comes home to eat and sleep. Without the emotional focus on the children, she and her husband are facing an empty nest. Nora wonders what is left of the passionate and intimate relationship they once had. Can it be rediscovered? Are there paths yet to explore on their journey or have they covered the globe already? Or, worse, has the last passion ship already set sail?

Jessie is an executive and a mother of two. She has often been chided for being a "closet prude." She makes flirtatious comments and sexual innuendos with the best of them, but beneath the surface she is really very embarrassed by the whole subject. She tolerates sex with her husband, feeling it is an obligation that she must bear. She will say that the thrill for her left after the first child was born. With her full-time career and two children, she professes to be too tired to care.

Jessie cannot even remember the last time she enjoyed sex with her husband. She says that when they do have sex, she does the "obligatory leg spread," closes her eyes, and sometimes throws in a few moans for effect. She adds, "He usually gets it over with pretty quick, thank goodness." Unfortunately, it sounds as if Jessie has given up or maybe never had it to begin with. It is true that Jessie has neither experimented nor tried anything "spicy" with her spouse. She was raised in a strict religious environment and claims this is the reason for her sexual inhibitions. To conclude that Jessie is a prude, however, is a superficial inference at best, for Jessie turns out to be a most enthusiastic participant in a quest for passion. Her sexual suppression eventually results in an explosion that rattles her moral and ethical beliefs to the core.

Carla, on the other hand, has had a lot of experience (and, yes, I mean sexually). She dated around, focused on her career, and waited until her forties to "settle down" and get married.

For a time, she was actually referred to by her friends as the Midwest's version of Samantha (after the promiscuous character on HBO's *Sex and the City*). By my standards, Carla's near three years of marriage qualify her as a newlywed, yet she is already feeling boredom in the bedroom. Carla is a corporate career professional who travels a lot for her job. She has been propositioned on just about every one of her road trips, usually by married men. Is Carla headed down infidelity lane?

Finally, there is Lisa. Lisa is a former executive, now a stay-at-home mom. She is very outgoing and an active community volunteer. Lisa talks a good game but has not participated in anything really wild — yet. During vacations, Lisa says, the sex is great, but once she and her mate are back home, making love becomes mediocre at best. Lisa has sought advice from every book she has gotten her hands on and has asked the advice of many a seemingly happy couple. A few times while she and her husband were on vacation, swingers (see "swinging" in the glossary at the back of this book) approached them. She is now very curious about the "lifestyle." With the goal of spicing things up, is Lisa heading toward "wild explorations"?

The stories of Courtney, Nora, Jessie, Carla, and Lisa are compilations of real events that happened to people who were willing to confide in me. I do not pass judgment on the actions of any of these people. In fact, I greatly respect them for finding their own way and for providing details of their lives and experiences, from which we can all benefit.

Through these women's journeys and the information and advice offered, we may get a glimpse of something we might want to try or something we wish to avoid. By sharing in these experiences, we may find our own way toward a more fulfilling and passionate sex life in our long-term relationship. Let the journey begin!

CHAPTER TWO

THE EXHAUSTED TRAVELER

PLACING A PRIORITY ON PASSION

In this chapter we take an in-depth look at our lifelong passion journey with our mate. We examine why watching the Travel Channel is not the same as being there. Going through the motions is never enough. We cannot put off "traveling" until we have the time and energy because that day will never come. Nor can we just wait at the terminal while the kids are growing up and hope our mate waits with us, because then we will miss all the flights.

We must decide whether our long-term relationship is going to be a luxury cruise or a third-rate traveler's nightmare. Do we want our mate there by our side throughout life's journey? Real-life stories in this chapter point out that some layovers, hassles, and delays on our journey are inevitable, and we have to put effort into dealing with them. Such effort requires placing a higher priority on our sexual and intimate relationship with our mate — with the ultimate of "travel" rewards.

IGNORE THE TRAVEL BROCHURES —
TAKE A JOURNEY TO REALITY

Do we have realistic expectations about passion in marriage? Long before reading romance novels as teenagers, many of us were dressing up as princesses, hoping someday to marry a handsome prince and live happily ever after. Romance novels, movies, soap operas, and even "reality" television shows do little to curb the romantic fantasy of a passion-filled life with Mr. Right. Of course, after we entered the dating world, reality started slapping us in the face. And after many years of dating and marriage, most of us believe we have a firm grasp on real life, recognizing that it is never going to be like it is in the movies.

However, these media images of passion-filled relationships have made an impact on our psyches. Sometimes we remember how promising the "travel brochure" looked and wonder why our marriage destination is not what we envisioned. Is there really such a thing as a passion-filled *long-term* relationship? Are there couples who know the secrets to keeping the spark alive long after the wedding bells stop ringing? Well, after researching passion in marriage, I have found many self-proclaimed happily married couples who, although they may not have "the answer," know many creative approaches and recognize one universal truth:

To keep the passion flame alive, we have to continuously feed the fire by placing a high priority on the intimate and sexual aspect of our relationship with our mate.

To accomplish this, we must first have realistic expectations. We cannot expect the passion to always sizzle — just as we cannot expect the passion to be there at all without putting time and energy into our sex lives. We may never have the fairy tale, but this does not mean we have to settle for the opposite extreme either. We know that "happily ever after" really means long-term work, effort, and commitment, and placing our relationship very high on the priority list, *especially* after the kids come along. This relationship priority includes cultivating intimacy through our sexual relationship. In other words, we cannot stay put. We must journey out, actively seeking and maintaining the passion in our relationship.

THE WEARY TRAVELER — HOW TO TAKE A JOURNEY WHEN WE WOULD RATHER TAKE A NAP

Audrey is like a number of women I know. After some years on the career path, she now stays home with her children. She is a go-getter in all that she does. Her days are very busy, filled with child care, laundry, dishes, errands, working out, soccer games, and the whole gamut of kid-related extracurricular activities. She does charity work, participates in church and social activities with other couples, and has extended family–related obligations. She is usually exhausted. Her husband is tired too, but especially tired of the fact that she expends all her energy on everything and everyone but him.

Don't get me wrong — Audrey is by no means ignoring her husband. She is following much of the latest pop psychology in "caring" for him. Audrey makes sure she is available to him whenever he is in the mood. She really has the best of intentions.

One night after dining out with friends, Audrey was tired but knew her husband wanted sex. She felt bloated and fat and completely put upon to come home exhausted and have to further "perform" for her mate. Her husband was angry. He was sick and tired of working so hard to support the family and receiving so little appreciation or pleasure for his efforts. He did not want Audrey to do him any favors. He wanted to feel as if she really wanted him and not that she was just fulfilling her wifely obligations.

Audrey was crushed. She knew he was right even though it was hard to hear the truth. Audrey had to admit that she rarely got into making love. It usually felt as if it was just another to-do to check off on her long list of chores. Her husband knew this. They had been together a long time. He recognized that she was just going through the motions. Audrey poured so much energy and passion into the roles of parent, housewife, friend, volunteer, and daughter. What happened to the energy and passion for the role of sexual partner?

Unfortunately, there are many people who do not recognize that the passion flame is dying in their relationship. Exhaustion and the constant feeling that there is too much to do are overwhelming, but are these good excuses for letting the passion flame expire? Is that project or that volunteer effort or that additional activity for the children or *any* of the extras really more important?

Sexual discontent in marriage is often cited as one of the top reasons for infidelity and divorce, so we must acknowledge the important role that making love plays in our relationship as a whole.

Audrey was recognizing that discontent in the bedroom was having a powerful and profound impact on her entire relationship. Her husband did not feel as if Audrey found him appealing anymore. He went so far as to say that he had a strong feeling she did not really love him anymore.

She prayed for guidance. As her marriage was obviously the foundation of her family, she intended to value it. So Audrey became determined to make no more excuses for her failure to find the energy. She very much wanted to feel the intimacy and the closeness that sex created with her husband — not to mention the sheer pleasure of it. And most important, she recognized that someday their children would be grown and would leave, but her husband hopefully would be there until death. She could not afford to let the passion continue to slip away.

And so we discover the first step of the journey . . . recognizing the importance of taking the journey itself. If we value the very foundation of our family — our lifelong mate — we will clearly see the importance of keeping the passion alive, of never placing our sex lives below the many to-dos that will hardly matter in the long run, let alone next week. The kids are too busy anyway and the dust will still be there, but will our relationship — with any depth — survive when the passion flame dies out? Will there be another opportunity or another day to relight it — or will it be too little, too late?

WHAT TO BRING ON THE TRIP AND WHAT TO LEAVE BEHIND

When we set out on a passion quest, we are seeking those moments when the excitement of his touch creates a hunger in us, and the intimacy fills us up. We are seeking the food that nourishes our relationship. We are seeking pleasure. We are seeking to fulfill our commitment to love and cherish. We are seeking the moments we will not forget. In recognizing what it is that we are seeking, we now have the best chance of finding it.

The journey will have many successes, if we start it off right. This means leaving the excess baggage behind and taking only that which will help us find our way. First and foremost we must leave behind that negative frame of mind.

Recently I was with a group of my girlfriends when Diane's phone rang. It was Lisa's husband calling to tell Lisa that he found her cell phone. Diane responded with a thank-you and told him that his wife loved him. Hearing this, Lisa said, "Do not tell him *that* — then he will think I want to have sex when I get home." We all laughed, but it made me pause and think. Why are we, as women, always complaining about sex with our mate as if it is a necessary evil in marriage? Why is our frame of mind toward the act of marital sex often so negative?

Whatever the reason, this negativity is baggage that we must leave behind on our quest for passion. We must pack instead a positive attitude. What if we suddenly, through death or injury, lost the opportunity to make love to our mate? If we love (or loved) our mate at all, we would come to regret the lost opportunities for those moments of intimacy and pleasure. We would desperately long to have that day back when we could have gone home and held him and made love.

So let us find a way to leave that negative baggage behind and pack what will make the journey a pleasurable one for years to come.

WHAT TO PACK FOR A PASSION QUEST AND WHAT TO LEAVE BEHIND

Leave Behind	Bring Instead
"Oh no, not again."	"All right! We get to do it again!"
"I better hurry and get to sleep before he comes to bed."	"I better hurry and get into my sexy nightie and light the candles before he comes to bed."
"Wish he would get this over with."	"Wish the pleasure would last longer."
All mental to-do lists.	Mental fixation on the sensation.
"If I do not move, maybe he won't realize I am still awake."	"If we make love, maybe I will be able to relax and get to sleep."
All thoughts of what is wrong.	Complete focus on what is right.
All focus on what he has not done.	Complete focus on what he does do.
Wishes that things were better.	Plans for making things better.

The excess baggage extends beyond all those negative thoughts toward sex with our mate. It includes the personal baggage that we bring into the bedroom — the reason for our exhaustion — taking on too much and trying to do it all. Furthermore, the personal baggage includes the image we carry of ourselves.

We will examine our self-image in later chapters, but its importance must be noted here. We have to do whatever possible to feel sexy — take better care of ourselves and fix ourselves up like we did when we were dating. We have to leave behind the baggage regarding our body image and our insecurities over our appearance.

Chances are our mate does not even begin to see all the flaws that we do when we look in the mirror. He is certainly not perfect either. If our mate feels loved and wanted, he will love us and want us back — and that really is all that matters. We women need to pay attention to the positive comments, focus on our gifts, and check negative-self-image baggage at the counter — and maybe, after we make love, we will forget to reclaim it.

PLANNING FOR OUR PASSION JOURNEY — THE ITINERARY TO PLEASURE

Once we are packed with only the necessary bags for our passion journey with our mate, we are set to venture out. It is time to really focus on making the quest a true success. Remember, we want the intimate, passionate aspects of our long-term relationship to be a luxury cruise and not have it turn into a third-rate traveler's nightmare.

To prevent the nightmare, the key is to plan ahead to avoid pitfalls and be prepared to manage those layovers and delays that will happen anyway. Sure, it would be easy and safe to never venture out at all — keep the status quo and let the safeness of mediocrity control our relationship. We may be comfortable with the way things are, but we also may be missing out on a lot of excitement, a lot of fun, and ultimately a lot of intimate moments of joy with our mate that will help keep us happily together.

As we create our itinerary to pleasure, we must work around the many factors that we are unable to control. For instance, we realize (at least, sometimes we realize) that we cannot control our mate. If we plan the itinerary with this in mind, we will find our way with much less frustration and heartache.

A good example of this is the story of Jane, a woman I met online through my Web site. Jane was complaining about how her mate was always unhappy with their sex life. She told me that he never put the moves on her anymore, and then he complained that they never had sex. I asked her if she ever initiated sex with him, and she replied with a question: "Why would I do that?" Apparently, as Jane explained it, if he really wanted her and desired her, then he would initiate the lovemaking. So, because he rarely put any effort into it, she assumed he did not want her and therefore had no right to complain.

I suggested to Jane that maybe her husband was feeling the same way that she was feeling. Maybe because she never initiated sex with him, he felt undesired and unwanted, and thought that *she* did not care enough to put a little effort into it. Someone had to take the initiative. I suggested to Jane that she end this standoff and take control of the situation by seducing him that night.

Jane's story highlights the fact that we all focus too much on how men and women are so different instead of focusing on how much we are alike. Men are also insecure, and they often need approval just as much as we do. A man's feelings of self-worth seem to depend heavily on sex and being sexually desired. It is inaccurate to say that making love is just a physical act for them. Men feel good about themselves when they feel desired — just as we do. By stepping into the bedroom arguments of couples such as Audrey and her husband, Jane and her mate, or the many people like them, we are able to recognize that this really is true.

> There is no grander way to show our spouse that he is appreciated and loved than to have passionate sex with him.

With this knowledge about men comes the power to make a difference in the relationship. We must recognize the important role sex plays in our relationship and use that knowledge to improve the situation. Do not wait for him to make the first move. Do not wait until it is too late. Right now, we have the power to show our love and appreciation in the most intimate way. We have the gift to nurture, caress, and create the environment wherein his needs *and* our needs have the best chance of being met.

The old adage is so true here — give and you shall receive. We are guaranteed to have an extremely pleasurable life journey with our mate if we focus on giving. I am not talking about this passion journey being akin to missionary work in the hot and bug-infested jungles of Southeast Asia. This is *not* self-sacrifice. I am suggesting that if we take charge and plan the itinerary, we will not only end up going where we want to go but also have a lot of fun getting there!

Planning the Itinerary — Choosing a Destination

If we wait, as Jane did, for our husband to make the first move, we might be waiting forever. It is not enough to simply want the passion to be alive in our relationship. To make the journey happen, *we* must plan the itinerary and choose the destination. When I lead group discussions about seeking the passion, I often discuss the necessity of taking the initiative in planning the "journey" and not rushing into anything without having mapped out the route. Taking charge of the passion quest in our relationship puts us in the driver's seat. We then have the power to take our mate to the sights that we want to see *and* make sure we arrive there safely.

In the coming chapters I will reveal the many creative routes that others like us have taken. Sometimes their stories and experiences will provide us with incredible ideas to expand our thinking toward sex with our mate. Sometimes their stories will reveal dangerous routes or dead ends that we may wish to avoid. By exploring these experiences, we will be better equipped to plan our journey and pick the "destinations" that work for our own relationship.

Planning the itinerary and choosing the destination does not mean focusing on the technique or particular mechanics of getting there. This is not a how-to about sex. A passion quest is about the bigger picture — where do we want our relationship to go? We do not want it to be stagnant. We want to feed the passion by seeking positive and creative destinations and avoiding those that will delay us or get us lost. In other words, because we want to travel with our mate for years to come, we want to plan a journey and set out on it with confidence that we are helping and not hurting our relationship.

Here, we are not going to consult the experts (sex therapists and the like). These "travel agents" may not have explored the far corners themselves. Without actual experience, they cannot describe the emotional impact and details of the real adventures that are being undertaken. However, we can make educated decisions when we have read the revelations of real-life women and their real-life efforts to rediscover passion and keep it alive. Then we go out and confidently choose the sights we wish to see and safely arrive at the destinations we wish to explore in our relationship.

The travel possibilities are endless, and what works for one couple may not work for another, but we can learn so much from the trials and tribulations of others. In examining the mistakes couples have made along the way, we can find a different route and avoid the pitfalls. By reading about what others have learned the hard way, we are able to plan a journey that is right for us and our mate, and are better prepared to find our own way toward a more passionate and fulfilling long-term relationship.

FREQUENT-FLIER MILES — EARNING OUR REWARDS

A well-thought-out passion quest has the promise of great rewards for our long-term relationship. Realistic expectations, placing a high priority on passion, and taking the lead to journey out will give us the best chance of getting quick and continuous rewards for our relationship as a whole. The alternative is to miss out on all the pleasures of the journey, all the frequent-flier miles . . . and will possibly result in the grounding of our relationship.

Will we someday be alone looking back on our long-term relationship and be full of regret? Will we wish we could take back the moments when we were too tired to care? What if our ability to function sexually wanes with age and our natural urges diminish — will we regret all those years we spent avoiding sex or rushing through it or putting off trying something new and creative? Will we regret not seeking the passion with our mate?

I certainly hope that will not be the case, especially since we have the power to do something about it. Someday I hope to look back on my marriage and fondly remember all the special, passion-filled moments I shared with my husband. I hope that he will be there next to me, holding my hand and smiling as we reminisce about our many passionate encounters together. We will have earned a lot of travel rewards. Our travelogue will not be full of regrets and missed opportunities but rather intimate moments, some exciting and others relaxing. Either way, they will certainly be worth remembering.

A passion quest for two is a vacation at home.

When we are on vacation with just our mate, we have a much better chance of detaching from the demands of children and work and extended family. We are able to focus on our mate and ourselves. The environment is conducive to romance, and we have an opportunity to relax and experience pleasure, both physical and emotional. Are we talking about an actual vacation? Of course that would be ideal, but most of us rarely get the opportunity to go away with just our mate. So we have to find this "vacation" right in our own home.

The people I have interviewed who put effort into creating passionate moments at home often *do* feel like they are away on vacation from the world, even when they are simply alone with their mate in their own bedroom. How do they accomplish this? We will answer that question in the coming chapters by examining the many ways couples utilize instinct, innate need, and creativity to reach their destination.

Some of the unconventional methods in later chapters illustrate not only the interesting and fascinating diversity in our culture but also the pitfalls and emotional injuries that can occur when people (accidentally or on purpose) venture out into unknown lands and explore the taboo. In reading about the fascinating and the extreme, we are able to recognize the reality of what some fantasize about and see the potential dangers to our relationship and to ourselves when fantasy becomes reality. We are also reminded of mainstream, tried-and-true methods that, when we apply them to our everyday lives, can reward us with many pleasures that we sometimes forget to find the time to enjoy.

Whatever we choose to take away with us from the stories I have collected, we must remember that we have chosen to take life's journey with our mate. Since we have booked the journey for two, we must not stay home alone, lag behind, get off at the wrong stop, or, worse, go off on our own. Any sincere and loving effort to journey out with our mate seeking to keep the passion alive comes with built-in travel insurance, and the rewards will be huge.

CHAPTER THREE

TRAVELING WITH OUR MATE

A CLOSER LOOK AT THE JOURNEY TOGETHER

WHY WE HAVE TO BE THE TRAVEL GUIDE

Whether it is in the many e-mails I get from my Web site or whether it is from my own support group, I am constantly hearing women complain about husbands that do not put any effort into making love. We often think maybe our spouse should get off his behind and put some thought and energy into romancing *us* again! Our mate sometimes seems to be the *king* of "wham-bam thank you, ma'am," and maybe without even any thank-you in there. This may be the case, but the question we need to ask ourselves is, *has complaining about it really helped improve the passion in our relationship?*

The same thoughts hold true for many men. In fact, I have received e-mails and inquiries on my Web site from males. They typically claim their mate does not really want any part of them anymore. They say she is often too tired for sex. Most express a strong desire for sex to become more of a priority in their relationship — "like it used to be." One man named Doug wrote the following: "It is like she does not care about me or my needs at all. Sure, she takes care of things around the house and cooks for me often, but when it comes to sex, it is just too big of a chore for her." Another man said to me, "She used to willingly make time for sex, but she rarely does so now — at least not with any enthusiasm." These comments reflect the widespread malady in long-term relationships. But again, I wonder, *has complaining about it really helped improve the passion in their relationship?*

The answer is usually a resounding *no!* Complaining or even just wishing he or she would change or do more has never gotten anyone anywhere. We all know this, yet we still complain and wonder why things never get any better at home. Well, the time has come for us to stop complaining and take action! Sometimes we are required to act as travel guide in our quest for passion. It is the only way to lead our mate where we really want to go.

We know that we cannot change our significant other. We have found that it is a complete waste of time to complain or to pressure our mate into putting more effort into making love. And, of course, it is fruitless to simply hope or wish the bedroom was heated like it used to be. Instead, research into real-life relationship success stories reveals that if we *make the effort* to please our mate and make him feel sexy and desired, this effort will have a huge payoff for us, and not just in the bedroom.

Taking the lead is empowering and allows us to choose the path that is right for us and our relationship. It puts the control in our hands and gives us the opportunity to make a difference. When we instigate change in our attitude and behavior, we have the power to change the relationship as a whole. We have found time and time again that the more we put into our sexual relationship, the more we get out of it. So, when we take the lead and guide him on a new path to passion, we will be creating a journey wherein our own needs have the best chance of being met.

> The more we put in, the more we get out. Or, the more we put out, the more we get out of it.

The "me first" attitude will not get us anywhere in our long-term relationship. We have to shed the "what has he done for me lately" attitude because it accomplishes nothing. After all, it is not our partner's responsibility to get us in the mood; we have to make an effort in that regard. What good will it do us if we are old and gray by the time we realize that we must take the lead to initiate change? It is far too easy to focus on what he is not doing for us, but an ultimately more productive solution would be to focus on what we could do for our mate. The best chance at motivating our partner to please us is to please him. Setting the example, taking our mate on the journey, and guiding him along the path is the fastest track to "Passionville."

If we feel the passion has left our bedroom, if we feel we have lost our way in our quest for passion, then we, as complex and creative people, must own the problem. And we have the power to solve it. We are the only ones with the ability to create the environment in which our needs may have the best chance of being met. Whether we are in bed with someone for the first time or the two thousandth time, we can create the mood we want and head down the path toward mutual sexual fulfillment.

THE MALE PASSION SEEKER'S VIEWPOINT

Many of the responses to the surveys on my Web site have been from men. These responses, coupled with interviews I have conducted, show clear and consistent support for the common belief that the act of sex itself is a very big part of emotional bonding for a man — for him to feel loved and appreciated in the relationship. The men tell us that their needs are arguably very simple, with the desire for sexual connection and satisfaction very high on the list. We women, on the other hand, believe we are a lot more complicated. High on our list are intimacy, emotional connection, and the need to be understood and, of course, romanced. Within these differences lies the problem.

The solution, though, is really quite simple. If we are to receive what we crave in our intimate relationships, *we* are going to have to make it happen. It is too easy to focus on what he is not giving us in our relationship or what he is not doing for us sexually. However, if we put the focus on what we are not doing for *him* and what *he* is missing, we now have the best chance to improve the situation for both parties. It is in the giving that we shall receive.

> If he truly feels sexy and desired in our eyes, he will feel loved and appreciated.

Frankly, the men could not be any clearer with us. They say it time and time again. "More sex, please" — and not just the "obligatory leg spread" but a genuine interest and enthusiasm for sex with him. It may very well come down to the idea that making a man happy in bed is making a man happy. If he truly feels sexy and desired in our eyes, he will feel loved and appreciated. This is what the men tell me and what I have many times found to be the case.

The husband of a friend of mine had one foot out the door in their relationship. He told me that when they were at their lowest point, he felt it was because she did not want to have sex with him anymore. He thought that if she loved him at all she would want to have sex with him, no matter what else was going wrong in their lives. His feeling of being unwanted permeated all aspects of their relationship. Slowly, through the input of her girlfriends' "passion quest support," his wife started putting some effort into their sex life again. The results were astonishing. Soon, the rest of their problems did not seem so overwhelming, and the intimate bond between them grew stronger again.

Of course, real-life problems do not evaporate just because we start putting effort into enthusiastically and creatively having sex again. However, when we are feeding the intimacy and the bond in our relationship, the tensions do ease a little. We may feel closer to our mate because the feeling of being alone or dealing with problems alone is reduced. And last but certainly not least, we are adding some fun and playfulness to our otherwise overworked life. All of this can go a long way toward helping both partners deal with the rest of life's issues.

Sadly, there are those times and those relationships in which no amount of effort seems to make a difference — the problems and the emotional disconnect are far too deep. There may be verbal and even physical abuse. In these cases, professional help becomes necessary. All our friends' advice, all the Passion Seekers' tips, and all the passion quests we can imagine are not going to solve anything. In these cases, there is no shame in seeking the help and professional assistance we need to find our way through it.

Even when the baggage is not overwhelming and the relationship is strong, mediocrity may still find its way into the bedroom — thus the point of a quest for passion. We must keep in mind that, when setting out on such a quest, making changes or even just suggestions can be a blow to that fragile male ego. (And who are we kidding? Our self-esteem is just as fragile.) His ego, especially with regard to his sexual abilities, needs to be stroked and encouraged. This seems particularly true when *we* take the initiative and set out to reignite the passion with our mate.

We all know that people like to be around those who make them feel good about themselves. Most men will tell us that they love having sex with someone who makes them feel as if they are a sexual master. They simply need to know they are great lovers. Criticizing and pointing out a man's sexual shortcomings in any way will not be productive. We can certainly understand this because so many of us feel the same way. If our mate complains about us sexually, we are certainly not encouraged to try harder to please him, in or out of the bedroom. On the other hand, when we are praised and encouraged, we are suddenly much more giving and appreciative.

If we focus on the positive and gush when something feels great, our mate will be encouraged. We can tell him what we love about his body, his touch, and his technique. We should constantly encourage him during sex and support his efforts. Most important, we can make suggestions through subtle means, taking care that our ideas do not come across as criticism of what he does do. We might try, for example, to incorporate what we would like him to do by working the suggestions into the details of a story we tell during sex — describing how hot such action would make us or our character in the story. Above all, we must find a way to assert ourselves and ask for what we want. This will give us a much better chance of getting what we need.

Once he feels our desire, once he feels we need and want him sexually, he will bend over backward to keep us satisfied, and not just in the bedroom.

Top Passion Seekers' Tips from the Men — Ways to Make Him Feel Sexy and Desired

(Note to the Guys: These Work for Her Too!)

- Initiate sex with your mate.
- Put some effort into looking sexy.
- Treat sex as a gift from your mate, not as a duty or chore.
- Exude tremendous enthusiasm for sex.
- Tune in to what your mate loves and generously supply it.
- Use your mouth all over him.
- Stroke more than just his ego.
- Think back to what you used to do for him that he really liked and do it again.
- Re-create the first time or take him on a second honeymoon.
- Have regular date nights and behave as if you are in date mode again.
- Just put a little effort into making love.

Taking the lead will result in him taking notice. We have consistently found that the efforts we start putting into our sexual encounters will encourage him to reciprocate. If we make him feel great, we will likely get the same in return. When he has been pleased, the standard of care we will receive will dramatically improve. So we should slip on a sexy attitude and go for it. Once he feels our desire, once he feels we need and want him sexually, he will bend over backward to keep us satisfied, and not just in the bedroom.

Overcoming Initial Roadblocks

Ultimately the efforts will pay off, but maybe not at first. It may take time. In fact, the initial attempts may not be well received. Any change in our behavior may bring questions from our mate and maybe even rejection. Although uncommon, there are occasions when our mate may feel threatened or intimidated by changes in the sexual-relationship routine.

I know someone who did not experience a positive response from her mate. She came into their bedroom one night in a sexy outfit, and her husband made fun of it. Another example came from a visitor to my Web site who said that her husband laughed at the "dirty story" she was trying to tell him during sex one night. Still another woman's husband thought that her new efforts meant she must be having an affair. Unfortunately, not all attempts to remedy a lack of effort in the bedroom will be accepted at first, but we cannot let this defeat our quest.

Through my surveys, interviews, and chats with my girlfriends, I have found several successful ways to ease into a quest for the missing passion by starting out with subtle changes. Some passion quests may require a slow departure, with more time spent in preparing for the adventure. In such cases, there are methods we can use to avoid having our efforts rejected *and* ways to handle the situation if our efforts are not well received.

Gradual Quest Departure Ideas

- Make sure you have done your "research" ahead of time. (See "Get Reacquainted with Your Travel Partner — Passion Seekers' Research Ideas" in chapter 9 of this book.)
- Set up a romantic date night — a candlelit dinner for two, etc., to set the mood.

- On the next birthday or gift-giving occasion, try giving him Passion Seekers' Coupons to use at *his* discretion (e.g., offering yourself in lingerie). Use the coupons in the back of this book or make up your own.
- If you do try a sexy outfit, you can give him advance warning by showing him the lingerie earlier in the day and offering to model it for him later, or better yet having him come with you to buy some new "bedroom attire."
- Leave him a little note or send him an e-mail at work to hint at what you are planning.
- Instead of telling him a story, first buy a book of erotica and read it to him.

There may nevertheless be times when the route we choose is rejected. Let's say he does laugh at our sexy outfit. We can choose to take this as rejection and get angry or we can laugh *with* him, and then grab him, kiss him, and threaten to take it off! Or we might threaten to tickle him to death and then proceed to do it. The point is not to take ourselves or him too seriously. We can choose to shrug the incident off and try again another night (give him and ourselves a rain check). We will look at the delay in our journey as a minor one. It might even be fun to view the situation as a seduction challenge and an opportunity to work a more intricate plan.

More likely than not, any and all efforts in the bedroom will not only be well received by our mate but result in a journey together to Passionville. Whatever we can do to show we care and appreciate our mate in bed will translate to goodwill in the relationship as a whole.

MY PET THE PENIS — CARING FOR THIS SPECIAL BREED

A large part of a successful quest for passion is understanding our mate's needs and, through our actions, placing a priority on meeting those needs. In the process, we will rediscover the passion in our relationship and in ourselves. So, for example, if we want to truly understand a man, it helps to look at our literal differences. One such difference is the penis.

Why do so many men so often complain about the lack of oral sex they receive? Why are their penises of such importance that they even name them? I have discussed the "penis issue" with my friends on many occasions. Then, armed with all our questions and ideas, I have opened the topic up for discussion at parties, in chat rooms, on my Web site, and through Internet surveys. As a result I have received quite an education, not from the so-called experts but from real people and real life. This is what I learned:

Imagine our sex organs are outside of our body, dangling between our legs, so fragile and vulnerable. Imagine — as a teenager or even as an adult — the embarrassment of a hard-on in public. Imagine the embarrassment of our mom discovering our sheets after a wet dream. Imagine the constant awareness we would have of our sex organs — adjusting them and protecting them. We have all seen otherwise strong, healthy men brought to their knees after being hit in the groin, watching them wither in excruciating pain with tears in their eyes. Imagine all of this as a backdrop, as we voyage toward a newfound appreciation of the male genitalia.

My Love Affair with a Penis

We may never fully understand the depth of importance men place on their penis, but the mere fact that they often speak of it, have an endless number of slang terms for it, and even actually name it should give us a clue. What would it be like if *our* sex organs were on the outside of our body? What would it be like if we could actually stimulate every inch of them *and* could actually feel with our hand and see the pulsating explosion of an orgasm? If we could do all this to the extent of our male counterparts, we just might begin to understand it.

So what does this mean to us? If we love a man and wish to continually have passionate sex with him, we will reap astonishing results by fully appreciating, loving, and even envying this amazing work of profound perfection that is the male genitalia.

Touch it, stroke it, play with it. . . . Love it like your pet!

One acquaintance of mine actually has a pet penis. Well, more accurately, she has a "pet penis philosophy." She often says that the key to a passionate relationship with a man requires only one approach: treat our mate's penis as if it were a house pet such as a dog or cat. Some of my friends and I (jokingly at first) put this philosophy to the test in what I refer to as the "pet penis trials." In this section, I will expand on the concept and reveal how this approach, as silly as it may sound, has been proved beyond the shadow of a doubt to be well received — even with the most sophisticated men.

The love and attention we put into our canine and feline friends translate into the perfect philosophy to apply to the passionate and intimate care of our mate. Let's look at it this way: how many times a day do we pet, cuddle, speak to, or otherwise pay attention to our dog or cat? We cuddle up on the couch with our pet. Many times a day, we pet, stroke, and scratch him in all the places he loves. What does our dog or cat give us in return? Complete love and adoration.

I suggest implementing the pet penis approach this way: Try for one week to treat your mate's genitalia as if it were your pet. Touch it every chance you get. Care for it and really show it love and affection, and not just in the bedroom as a prelude to sex. In the morning before you get out of bed, in the bathroom, when you are sitting on the couch, under the kitchen table during meals, even in public (discreetly brushing up against it), pay attention to it during the many moments throughout the day — like you would your pet. At the end of the week you will be astounded by the ample return on your investment.

Proper Care and Feeding of Our Pet

> As with our dog or cat, our attentions to our pet penis will result in *special devotion to us,* as its primary caretaker.

Caring for our pet and keeping it healthy is necessary to ensure its continued availability and devotion to us. If we ignore our pet for days on end, merely going through the motions, our pet will suffer and perhaps even run off. If we just put out a little food and water but never talk to, care for, or stimulate our pet, what will happen? Our pet may become lazy or naughty. It might get extremely moody and agitated. It will certainly be less inclined to provide us with the love and adoration we so desire!

In the bedroom, we can frequently give our pet a treat — it is *healthy* for this kind of pet to get fat — and as a result it may even do tricks for us! We especially need to pay attention to our pet even when sex is not the ultimate goal. During sleep time or after making love, we can cuddle up to our pet penis, stroke and caress it, kiss it, and otherwise show it affection. As we drift off to sleep, we can hold it or just put our hand on it. A true and honest appreciation for our pet penis will reap great rewards. As with our dog or cat, our attentions to our pet penis will result in *special devotion to us,* as its primary caretaker.

We will also learn a great deal about our pet if we pay close attention to it. Even if we have had our pet for many years, it is to our advantage to take inventory from time to time — simply because things never stay the same. Where does our pet particularly like to be stroked? What makes our pet grow larger? What makes our pet squirm? What makes our pet really sit up and pay attention to us? Soon we may fully appreciate what makes our pet really happy. With this knowledge comes power — the power to control our pet and the power to utilize it to our advantage, or perhaps I should say *satisfaction.*

This pet penis philosophy may sound like a witticism to some, but it is offered to illustrate an important point: providing intimate attention to our mate keeps us on the path of a sincere, loving, and passionate relationship quest. If we give our mate attention and affection and thereby create a fun and loving environment, not only will our mate be happier and feel more appreciated but we will have created an environment in which our own needs have a better chance of being met. An appreciated spouse is much more apt to provide us with love, affection, and many passionate moments — moments that remind us how lucky we are to be sharing our life with someone special!

CHAPTER FOUR

CREATIVE EXPEDITIONS

SEX AS A FORM OF ART — PASSION SEEKERS' TIPS

Nora and her husband, Bob, were finding that their children were not distracting them much anymore. Nora's eldest (and only daughter) had just left for college, and Nora's son was rarely around these days. The atmosphere around their home was evolving. Nora and Bob had managed to stay together through so much — which was no small feat — and they were now facing an opportunity to really focus on each other again.

With this focus came the realization for Nora that their quests for passion had for quite some time become quick trips to the local convenience store instead of explorations of new and exciting destinations. She could not recall the last time that a quest with her husband had really rocked her world. Besides,

what was really left to explore? After twenty-some years of marriage, they had pretty much tried everything or at least everything they were willing to try — or so Nora thought.

Nora and a group of her female friends were always looking
for a fun excuse to get together. Nora laughed when I told her
about the pet penis philosophy, but she immediately agreed to
host a Passion Seekers' party. With Nora facing a near-empty
nest, she told me she was more than ready to put some focus on
her long-term relationship, and taking a journey to seek the missing passion was just what she had in mind.

The very first evening with Nora and her friends provided all
of us with a refresher in "creative expeditions" (see glossary at
the back of this book). Nora's friends each showed up with a
bottle of wine and lots of attitude. They all had strong opinions
that were initially expressed with knowing glances and frequent
rolling of the eyes, but soon we moved the conversation away
from the typical male bashing and on to something more productive. I asked each person to give me her best advice on how
to get one's love life back on track and re-create passion in the
bedroom. As we emptied the wine bottles, the list grew long and
the ideas more creative and inspiring.

Clearly none of these fortysomething and fiftysomething
women had lost any interest in sex. In fact, they were finding
that they had more time now to take a passion quest and were
looking forward to many new adventures. Even Nora was beginning to express hope that she and Bob could create or re-create
the *fun* again. The consensus was that "traveling" is always an
adventure when we keep an open mind and try something
new — or at least revisit a long-forgotten "location."

The scenario at Nora's first Passion Seekers' party has since
been played out time and time again. Opening up with girlfriends reminds us of the possibilities for creativity in the bed-

room and inspires us to rekindle the passion in our long-term relationship — whether we have been with someone three years or twenty-three years or even more.

It was with Nora's group that my education on creativity began. Just what can *we* do to produce new adventures at home? I have since asked this question of scores of women who have been traveling with their mate for many years. It is from the real-life experiences of people in the trenches of long-term relationships that we receive the best advice. Many of us, including those who have gone through divorces and other such losses, are able to offer universal inspiration and creative ideas and tips from which we can all benefit. Maybe we have already "been there and done that," but in the sharing, we are reminded of the fun and exciting journeys that await us if we just put a little renewed effort into producing at-home adventures.

Nora is the perfect example. From boredom and "quick trips" to creative and passionate expeditions, Nora eventually came full circle in her relationship — a return to the days of waiting for him at the door and not even making it to the bedroom before they took their clothes off. With the focus returned to her long-term relationship came the opportunity and the promise of new adventures awaiting her and her long-term mate.

Nora's passion quests became something to look forward to again and brought a renewal to the second half of her marriage. How this happened was really quite simple. Nora once again put effort into producing intimate and passionate moments, and found a new creative outlet that even inspired her mate. Her ability to do this came from remembering the details again. It came from chatting and sharing with other women. It came from the motivation to have a marriage that wasn't as empty as her nest was becoming.

CREATING AT-HOME ADVENTURES

When my curiosity about passion in long-term relationships surfaced (after having children and experiencing many years of marriage), I found that people love to have an excuse to talk about sex. At first, the talk may not always be about the person's own sex life, but eventually personal details come out. My best sources have come not only from Passion Seekers' parties but also from conversations with total strangers, especially in the anonymous atmosphere of a vacation resort. As we will find through Lisa's adventures in chapter 9, people on vacation tend to be more relaxed and in the party mood. This is a perfect time to discuss sex, because the subject is often a favorite topic of conversation anyway.

So what do these conversations reveal about sex and passion in a long-term relationship? They show us that the possibilities for sexual variety — even at home alone with our mate — are endless. These titillating ideas will hopefully act as stimulants (figuratively and literally) to get our creative juices flowing.

We do not have to go somewhere exotic or be with someone exotic — wild experiences between spouses are happening right in our neighborhood bedrooms. Having great sex time and time again comes from creating a certain mind-set and mood, and exhibiting a little enthusiasm. To do this, we must break out of our routine. Accepting that we all have sexual needs that are as basic as our need for food and water is just the beginning. We have to train our mind to think of sex as a form of art in which our creativity may be released and blossom. We must create the scene. We are the performer, the director, and the producer. If we take the lead, we are then in control and have the power to make a difference in the bedroom.

To take the lead in creating that passion again and again, we must paint a picture or compose a song in our mind and release that feeling into our creation. We all have the power to create, and in the act of creating, we are energized. Our sexual desires will increase tenfold as we adjust our mind to think of the act of sex as a masterpiece, begun anew each and every time.

Feeling too tired is a common problem for us all. We are overextended. However, if we set up the scene and initiate the play, we will become inspired and energized. Repeatedly, after discussing, researching, or writing about passion and sex, I have found that, when the time comes, the inspiration is always there. As a writer, I know that simply sitting down at the computer and typing the mind's ramblings can result in the beginning of a great story. The same holds true for sex. Our inspiration may come from an evening with our friends, talking, laughing, and confiding in one another about sex. It may come from a romance novel. Or it may come from something as simple (and important) as recognizing that our partner in life needs to know that we appreciate and care for him. Fortunately, nature has provided us with the perfect, most natural way to express that appreciation — intimately and passionately alone together.

And so we must begin. Take the lead and start the play in motion. The inspiration will come and the energy will surface. The show is bound to be a success. The key is to never act out the same play twice — and this chapter explains just how to do this. The ideas of real people with real-life examples will help us expand our thinking and attitude toward sex, and help us open the vast realm of creative possibilities that exist within the confines of our sexual relationship with our partner.

The key is to never act out the same play twice.

No matter how long we have been with our partner, it is very likely that we have only begun to realize the depth of our partner's sexual fantasies, not to mention our own. Our fantasies are ever changing, and the variations are endless. If we try, we can conjure up images in our mind and visualize a hot sexual encounter. The goal is to tap in to both our own *and* our partner's imagery and utilize these thoughts in our next physical encounter.

Communication of sexual fantasies can be a land mine. But if our sexual relationship has become routine, it is time to shake things up and risk an explosion. This is not the time to tread lightly. We must take a chance and break out of our comfortable sex routine by using our imagination to create a variety of moods, scenes, and fantasies in the bedroom.

We have found that it is all too easy to get into the habit of using the same maneuvers that have worked in the past. Maybe they still "work" and achieve orgasms, but we are missing the excitement of something new and different. The act becomes a rerun. We should strive instead to produce a new show, and not just once or twice. Every time the curtain goes up, we must play the part a little differently. Remember, we have the power to not only star in the lead role but direct and produce the show as well. Some of the best advice in the "business" follows:

The Lady and the Tramp

To initiate a production of a new sort, we begin with a variety show. For example, on the first night, we create a "nasty" mood. Before we are even alone with our mate, we call him up at work early in the day and tell him that he has been naughty and is going to be "punished" tonight. He will anticipate and think about it all day. After work or while doing chores, we'll be playful with him. We can swipe him on the butt, spray him with water, or surprise him with a pinch on his nipple. It is a good idea to start with a little playful naughtiness, and then accelerate it in the bedroom. Now, behind closed doors, we can teach him a lesson he will not forget. We will not be tender or loving. We will not whisper sweet nothings. Instead we'll tell him what he must do as his punishment. When was the last time we told him we wanted to be f—ked? We'll do it, go with it, play the part and do what feels right. Maybe we will really have to act at first, but soon we will not be acting; we will be living the part.

However, the next time, we can play out a completely different scenario. This time we will be a lady and make love. We'll leave him a note in his briefcase or an e-mail on his laptop expressing how much we appreciate him and listing what we love about him. We all too often tell our husbands what they do wrong or what they forget to do and rarely positively reinforce the good. So on this day and night, we will play the role of the adoring wife by loving him tenderly, using candles and slow music, or just being soft and inviting. We can try a massage and sensually spoken words, slowly complimenting whatever is physically appealing about our partner. At the same time, we can drag out the touching to the point of exasperation, with long leisurely strokes with the tongue and fingers.

> If we let ourselves, we will *become* the role and will be carried away by it.

Whether we act the lady or the tramp or a combination of the two, we must create the image in our mind and envision the role. We should go for an Academy Award. The more we get into the part, the hotter the scene will become. Props and scenery are helpful, but the only real tool we need is our mind.

We will feel sexy if we establish the image in our thoughts and focus on playing it. Soon we will not be acting the part at all. If we let ourselves, we will *become* the role and will be carried away by it. We have nothing to lose and everything to gain — inside and outside the bedroom. The reward will be not only the approval and admiration of our mate but his satisfaction and ours as well.

Romantic Versus Frantic

Changing the pace of sex is another favorite way to add variety to the "show." There is a lot to be said for "fast and frantic." Maybe we need to be in the mood before fast and frantic will happen for us. Again, we can find that mood by creating it in our mind. We might read an erotic book or romance novel, or see a sexy movie. Then, when we feel the heat, instead of waiting for the end of the chapter or the movie, we must find our partner and rip his clothes off.

Passion Seekers have many favorite sexy books and movies. A selected list is provided at the back of this book. Personal favorites include the romantic historical novels by Jo Beverley. She has a way of creating a passionate mood in her stories that will stimulate and invigorate without being explicit. Sources such as this will help to remove our thoughts from the day's responsibilities. Fifteen minutes of such reading each day can get us in the right frame of mind and can do wonders for our ability to passionately approach our mate.

An alternative to fast and frantic is the "formal date approach." We must not wait for him to set up a date with us. We will make the reservations, find a sitter, and buy a sexy outfit or a new pair of shoes. The pace of the formal date approach is slow and intimate. We might have a glass of wine. We'll touch him any time we can, *all evening long.* We will kiss every moment we can, just like we did on those early dates. The key is to build the anticipation. On the ride home, we'll whisper in his ear, touch him, and pet him. Then, once at home, we will slowly take off his clothes and then slowly take off ours. We'll make out with our mate, kissing our way down and giving him some intimate loving.

> The efforts we put into exploring the spectrum of possibilities will inspire our mate.

The pace, just like the style, can be altered from one night to the next, or we can do a little of both in one show. The point is to mix it up and find a wide range of scenarios. The efforts we put into exploring the spectrum of possibilities will inspire our mate. We will then be inspired to create new scenarios together. Playing off each other and taking cues from our mate will result in a new production.

Sound Effects

Every great performer knows how to use his or her voice effectively. Our voice has a powerful and profound impact on the person we love. To utilize this to its fullest, we must add variety in the way our voice creates the mood in the room. Sexy compliments breathlessly uttered, telling him what is hot about him and what he is doing right, will go a long way toward setting the mood and reassuring him that he is on the right path. With such reassurance, he will recognize the fact that we are enjoying the moment and are happy to be having relations with him. When he feels truly loved, he will naturally feel gratitude. He will become more giving and more eager to please us.

We can vary the use of our voice with lots of sexy talk on one occasion and then no talk at all on the next — just pleasurable moans, breaths, and sighs. On yet another occasion, we can tell him a story. As set out in "Story Time, Fantasyland, and Imaginary Playmates" later in this chapter, storytelling is another great technique that allows us to use our voice to add variety and passion to our long-term lovemaking.

The Role of a Lifetime

The roles people play when creating variety in the bedroom vary far beyond what will be touched on in this book. The BDSM (bondage, discipline, sadism, masochism) information set out in chapter 8 notwithstanding, we have all heard of the many dominant versus submissive bedroom games for husbands and wives to play. The common, tamer versions include the usual pairings of doctor and nurse, hotel guest and French maid, pool boy and housewife, teacher and student, and boss and employee (see more complete list below). Props can add a lot to these sorts of role-playing games. To broaden the spectrum of fun and fantasy in our long-term relationship, the possibilities should be explored with an open mind. We should do what feels right and remember the ultimate goal: an intimate and passionate relationship full of "that feels great" moments.

Passion Seekers' Role-Playing Ideas

- doctor — nurse or patient
- pool boy — housewife
- teacher — student
- boss — employee
- firefighter — victim
- master — slave
- hotel guest — French maid
- gardener — homeowner
- military officer — enlistee
- hooker — client
- warden — prisoner
- jock — cheerleader

- police officer — suspect or detainee
- knight — damsel in distress

- celebrity — fan
- judge — juror

Remember, what works one night will not necessarily work the next — for either partner. To become routine in our lovemaking is to become boring and eventually ineffective. The variety we create is what will keep our sex lives forever interesting. We have found that even just adjusting our attitude to be open to all the options will set us on the road to a more passionately fulfilling long-term relationship.

Ten Ways in Ten Days

Sometimes our routine just needs a little kick in the butt. A workout buddy of mine once recommended a marathon experiment. She said to try different methods of making love every night for ten days — ten ways in ten days. Alternatively, a mini-marathon might do the trick — sex every day for five days. Either way, no matter how tired we are or busy or otherwise uninterested, we will just "do it" every day regardless. We may find that at the end of the set period we are actually craving sex more often. It might just jump-start a new creative sexual life with our mate. Breaking out of the routine of sex once a week or every Saturday or even every few days will help to create that new and passionate environment we crave.

STORY TIME, FANTASYLAND, AND IMAGINARY PLAYMATES

Learn to Tell a Great Story

One of the greatest mood-enhancing techniques out there, repeated to me time and time again, is to tell our mate an erotic story during foreplay and sex. It will focus not only his mind but ours as well. Telling a story forces the day's responsibilities out of our mind and puts us in the moment. We then have the control to take him where we want to go. It is our voice dancing around in his mind. The images we are creating are the visions in his mind. We are sharing the fantasy with him.

Some women I have interviewed initially expressed concern over coming up with a sexy story, professing to not be creative enough or feeling silly about it. In these cases, I recommend using "story starters." There are several ways to do this. One way is to ask our mate, during foreplay or a massage, to start a sexy story about a fantasy of his. Then we take over with seductive details and elaborate on the "action." We can act some of it out and encourage him to do the same. We can also involve imaginary others in the action to create a fantasy in our own bedroom — a fantasy that both partners can share together.

When people continue to have trouble creating "story talk" in the bedroom, I suggest using a previously written story (see "Passion Seekers' Author and Magazine Picks" at the back of this book for ideas). We can read the sexy story in the book or magazine to our mate while he is massaging us or touching us. Then we can finish the story our own way, either expanding on it or elaborating as things get hot.

Passionate Journeys of the Mind:
Some Possible Story Starters

START EACH ONE WITH "IMAGINE . . ."

- we sneak into their bedroom during the party and . . .
- that time when you and I were . . .
- I lock the door to your office and open my coat . . .
- we are lying on the beach, looking at the stars, when she approaches us . . .
- we are hiking in the woods when we come upon a couple that is . . .
- when the room-service attendant arrives, I take off his/her uniform while you watch us . . .
- I am in the closet, watching you touch her . . .
- you are in the closet, watching me take his clothes off . . .

As we will see in chapter 9, some research about our mate's preferences is important. It is, of course, necessary to gauge which fantasies are best kept to ourselves or at least modified somewhat. A little discussion beforehand, through the use of erotic literature, etc., is helpful. Many times, for men, the more detailed and pornographic the story, the better. Remember, amazingly enough, as we are forced to focus on the sexy events we are describing, the thoughts of the laundry and other such responsibilities are pushed clear out of our mind.

We Are Now Entering Fantasyland

One Passion Seekers' party resulted in the revelation of a great bedroom secret — that of incorporating imaginary play-mates into lovemaking. It is human to have erotic thoughts and fantasies about others. As Dossie Easton and Catherine Liszt say in *The Ethical Slut,* "A ring around the finger does not cause a nerve block to the groin." This is reality, and it is better if we just accept it. However, realizing that we still fantasize about others does not mean we have to carry out the fantasy. For some, acting on these feelings (in an up-front manner) is considered okay, but for many this is not the case. In fact, we will see in coming chapters the assorted hazards involved with living out such fantasies. So as long as we "come home to eat," does it really matter where our appetite comes from?

With the use of imaginary playmates, not only will he come home to eat but his appetite, as well as ours, will be created through the use of our imagination. This approach goes arm in arm with storytelling. It entails the following:

First, we have to be open to venturing into fantasyland. Just as we have images at play inside our head whenever we make love, our mate has similar thoughts. It can be a lot of fun to share these images and thereby feed off each other's sexual imagery. These fantasies that either partner conjures up in the bedroom are just that — fantasies, creative images. He is still there with us, enjoying our body and no one else's. So why not share what is already going on inside both partners' heads anyway? Why not share the fantasy together? Having shared these intimacies, we will ultimately feel even closer to our mate, as opposed to wondering what is going on inside his head when he is making love to us.

With that in mind, we can invite an imaginary playmate into the bedroom. For instance, we will describe for our partner what this playmate is doing to us or what she is doing to our partner. We can also show him. Better yet, we can describe to our mate what *he* is doing to this playmate, creating the image in his mind that we are this other person. We will tell him what to do to her. As our mate is making love to us, we will describe it to him as if he were doing it to this playmate. We may tell him we like watching what he is doing to her and that she is enjoying it. There are many sexy directions we can go with this.

Inviting imaginary playmates into our bedroom gives us a sort of mind control. We are creating the scene and the images that are now dancing around in his head. We are setting the sexy mood while at the same time adding variety to the event. The mind control applies to us also. We can all remember times when, while making love with our mate, we were thinking about some project at work, some mess downstairs, or some other matter. Instead of putting ourselves in the position of letting our mind wander off the subject and on to our worries, we can use the story to keep our mind focused. While we are telling the story and describing the playmate, our mind is also focusing on the moment, the touch, the imagery, and the action. The use of stories and imaginary playmates will get us into the game and keep us focused on the moment.

LOCATION, LOCATION, LOCATION!

A favorite topic among Passion Seekers is "location sex." Some of us have great stories from our dating years and early on in our marriages about different places we have made love. However, since the years have passed and the children have come along, the variation on location has in many cases come to a screeching halt. With the exception of vacation sex, most of us cannot drum up any recent memories of anywhere unusual that we have made love.

The exception is Tonya. Tonya is a "pro" at what we call "party sex." During the course of whatever party they happen to be attending, she and her husband have sex in the bathroom.

Her theory is that when her desire is peaking (say after two glasses of wine), that is the time to go for it. Waiting until late at night after getting home, dropping off the babysitter, and readying for bed doesn't work — they are too tired and the energy and heat are gone. Her friends have learned to help themselves to additional refreshments if Tonya and her husband are both missing at a party at their house. Tonya's tips: always make sure the door is locked, and go to a remote bathroom so that an impatient line does not interrupt you.

One evening, the Passion Seekers brainstormed about unusual places to have sex. We all vowed that by the next month we would make love to our mate in an unusual location, somewhere other than our bedroom. Missy's choice was her husband's office. She had made plans with her husband to pick him up at his job to take him out to lunch. Missy showed up in her coat and high heels and *nothing* else. She surprised her husband with "lunch," "Brazilian style" (see glossary at the back of this book). Her husband was so thrilled and excited by the event that he calls her regularly to ask for his lunch to be delivered "Brazilian style."

For some reason we recall sex in a parked car when we were young as hot and passionate. Now the word that comes to mind is "uncomfortable." Thus we have found the real purpose of a luxury sedan or large SUV. Believe me, friends, the mere suggestion that he is going to get laid in an SUV just might cinch the sale of the larger luxury model. Additionally, we have found that police officers are typically much more understanding when a couple over thirty-five is caught having sex in a parked car when the pair tells him that the marriage counselor suggested it. But a word of caution: this excuse works only if one is actually with one's spouse.

Hotel sex is a location favorite. Although we are at risk of having ordinary "vanilla sex" (see glossary at the back of this book) as easily at a hotel as at home, there is something special about a hotel room. Nora, for example, has decided that this is the best place for role-playing games (see "Passion Seekers' Role-Playing Ideas" listed in this chapter). She checks in alone, then "picks up" her husband, Bob, in the hotel bar. Sometimes Nora has him deliver "room service." She also highly recommends the use of a condom, claiming it feels different that way and helps with the role-playing.

When the weather is nice, we might try slipping out into a tent in the backyard in the middle of the night or, if we have some privacy in our backyard, trying what my friend Mila suggests. Mila and her mate love to slip out naked into their backyard and have sex. She insists it is the next best thing to making love on the beach. She is a big fan of the moon and stars as mood lighting. The sounds of nature and the breezes and the cool night air provide added atmosphere. Mila insists, though, that complete nudity is a necessity because it feels free and natural and puts her more in touch with her "animal instincts."

If we are stuck with "doing it" (again) in the master bedroom, the Passion Seekers suggest we make it "fantasy location sex." This concept, used regularly by many visitors to my Web site, involves creating a place in our mind and orally describing the scene to our mate, thus bringing him with us. (For some, a blindfold or mask is helpful.) One example is using a romantic place we have visited. At the time we were at this location, perhaps we wished we could have "done it" right there or were otherwise turned on at that moment. We can describe the place in detail. If there is music associated with the location, we can put that music on. If there are smells such as suntan lotion or fragrant flowers, we can re-create that as well. Through our descriptions, we will put ourselves and our mate there. We can describe what we did to him as we do it again — or what we would have done to him if we could have. We can go there in our mind and bring him with us. Fantasy location sex is a great tool to use if we need to get our mind into the moment and the mood.

Another option is to give our mate a bath or a shower, or invite him into ours. There is a reason that the shower is one of the top places in which men and women masturbate. The shower is often forgotten as an excellent, relaxing location to even just initiate the process of making love. We do not have to wait until he comes to bed. Instead we can take advantage of the heat and the steam and the caresses of the water flowing down our sudsy naked flesh. We can use our hands and soap him up all over. My tip is to try different aromatherapy body washes for added sensory overload or, for a tub or Jacuzzi, use those scented candles that rarely get lit.

When all else fails, we can use a chair. The chair itself is a location because of the position possibilities (we are talking about a regular armless chair). Try a boss-and-secretary story or other such role-play.

Passion Seekers' Locations *Not* to Seek

- Airplane bathrooms. They are just too damn small these days and they always stink. As an alternative, some airports have very nice individual bathrooms or phone rooms in the airline members-only lounges. However, if you are really set on sex in the sky, go to milehighclub.com to find out how to "earn your wings" in comfort — one couple I met "highly" recommends it.
- The locker rooms at the country club (or the gym, for that matter). This is an issue only if you value your club membership (even if they do not throw you out, you will be whispered

about). However, some clubs have janitor closets that are infrequently used and are a safer bet than the locker rooms.

- The woods without a blanket or sleeping bag. The odds are
slim of actually finding a spot comfortable enough for *both* of
you to actually achieve orgasm.
- Church. For obvious reasons. (By the way, if you are ever
speaking to my priest, everything suggested in this book is for
the purpose of procreating.)

Mentioned a few times already is one of the very best locations for great, passionate marital sex — vacation. Time and
time again, when researching and uncovering great sex stories, I
heard from married couples who recounted events from their
vacation. I absolutely insist that if there is only one thing we do
differently with our mate after reading this book, it is to take a
vacation alone with him at least once a year. It can be something
as simple and brief as a weekend getaway, camping in the woods,
or even just playing tourist in our own city while staying at a nice
hotel. Of course, the best plan, if we are able, is to get away for a
whole week and go somewhere exotic. (A fabulous book of great
and sexy adults-only locations and vacations is *Adults Only
Travel: The Ultimate Guide to Romantic and Erotic Destinations*
by David West and Louis James.) Whatever our choice, we have
to escape from the children and the many responsibilities at
home and give our relationship some fresh air. This does not
include going on vacation with a group of other couples because
the dependence on our mate is lost and the chance of intimate
conversations and romantic encounters is greatly decreased.

Many couples I have met swear that a sexy vacation with our
lifelong mate can carry us the whole year. For example, Lisa and
her husband start getting excited about their upcoming vacation

each spring, a month or so before they are to depart. They work out together more often. Lisa starts shopping for sexy outfits — clothes she would never be caught dead in at the country club. She models them for her husband. The "anticipation sex" is great.

Then, at the resort, Lisa and her husband play lots of sexy games. Often Lisa's husband is the photographer and Lisa is his model. They have photo shoots and run back to their room for "wardrobe changes" (and, of course, other activities). It adds fun and excitement to act like someone else for the week or just to cut loose — flirt, act silly, lie out naked, and really enjoy each other. It also helps to treat each moment of our vacation as if we are on a date with our mate for the first time — keeping our makeup on, closing the bathroom door when we are using the toilet, and flirting with him!

For months after Lisa and her husband return from vacation, they have great sex by reliving the memories, re-creating the mood in their bedroom, and remembering how great it is to be living their life with someone special. With a positive and creative attitude toward vacation alone with our mate, we may just find that "passion pot of gold" at the end of the rainbow.

Of course, we are often without the luxury of a childless vacation with our mate. When that is the case, we have to get a little more creative in making our passionate moments happen with our partner. One acquaintance of mine recommends "amusement park foreplay." This entails a conscious effort to be playful all day, and not with our kids. We can try the pet penis approach (see chapter 3) in a discreet fashion — such as touching on dark rides. We can kiss him often and even hold hands. Not only will it be great for our children to see (appropriate) affection between both partners but our actions will serve as foreplay for later when the kids are asleep. Children never sleep more soundly than after a day at an amusement park.

Nora and her friends suggest that if we find ourselves with an empty nest — either temporarily or when the kids have moved out — we should rediscover the rest of our home and explore our town. Perhaps we remember, from our dating years, going to the zoo, on a picnic, or to an amusement park. We need to try exploring like a kid again. We can plan a day touring in our hometown on a date with our mate. We might try going somewhere new or just seemingly new because we are now free of children. It is fun to take pictures of each other, discuss the sights, and continually touch him. Then, when returning home to that empty nest, we should consider that now anywhere in our home can be the boudoir. We can turn off the lights, light candles around the house, walk around in lingerie, and make love in every room of our home.

All the location ideas mentioned in this chapter have been effective and useful for real people, just like us, who are hoping to keep the passion alive in their long-term relationship — and are actively and successfully doing just that.

Creative Expeditions

This chapter reminds us of (or opens our eyes to) the possibilities for passionate expeditions. They are endless. All we need to do is utilize our creativity — that same talent we have for decorating our house or making a Halloween costume or throwing a great party or planning a project at work. We simply need to apply it to our most important relationship.

The Passion Seekers' Dozen —
Creative Expedition Pointers

- Think of the act of sex as a form of art in which your creativity may be released.
- Take the lead for a change and run the production your way.
- Create variety by sometimes making love as the "lady" and sometimes playing it nasty as the "tramp."
- Alternate the pace — sometimes fast and frantic and sometimes slow and romantic.
- Use a variety of sound effects, including sexy compliments breathlessly uttered, pleasurable moans and sighs, and nasty encouragements.
- Consent to a power exchange — select a role to play from the chart in this chapter.
- Jump-start the passion with a marathon "Ten Ways in Ten Days."
- Tell a dirty story — use the list of story-starter ideas in this chapter.
- Invite an imaginary playmate into the bedroom.
- Venture outside the bedroom and seek unusual locations.
- Take a vacation with just your mate to a romantic and exotic location.
- Fully utilize your creativity and seek a new and different quest every time.

Remember, sex with our long-term mate is an art form in which our individual creativity may be released and blossom. The real-life ideas set out in this chapter will hopefully inspire us to create our own production. Taking the lead and putting some renewed effort into our intimate relationship will inspire and motivate our mate. The journey of creative expeditions will take our relationship to new, unexplored heights. Happy trails!

CHAPTER FIVE

PERILOUS JOURNEYS

TO STRAY OR NOT TO STRAY

Despite the endless variety of creative expeditions that we may explore alone with our mate, there are couples out there who do not buy into the societal prescription of conventional monogamy. They have found ways to lead their lives with long-term relationships full of love, sex, intimacy, and companionship, but without sexual monogamy. Some swingers have managed to stay emotionally committed to their long-term relationship while sharing with their partner in new sexual exploits with outsiders. In other types of nonmonogamous relationships, referred to as "open relationships," the couple agrees that each person on his or her own may be sexually and even intimately involved with people outside the relationship.

When talking with people involved in these various alternative sexual lifestyles, I found that they all say essentially the same thing: our society's idea of marriage simply does not work. They point out that of the approximately 50 percent of couples in the United States who actually stay married, many are unhappily married and many are having affairs — emotionally, physically, or both (see "The Current Estimates for the United States" in chapter 1). They all express a strong belief that their lifestyle — whether involving an open relationship, swinging, or some other alternative that allows for sexual exploits with someone other than their partner — is by far a more honest and natural approach to a relationship, as opposed to sexually repressing their desires and deceiving their partner and themselves.

There are several books, some focusing on the emotional perspective and some focusing on the scientific, that describe the many studies "proving" that humans are not naturally monogamous. Therapist and author of *The Monogamy Myth* Peggy Vaughan states, "Monogamy is not the norm. Society gives lip service to monogamy but actually supports affairs." Behavioral scientist David P. Barash and psychiatrist Judith Eve Lipton assert in their book *The Myth of Monogamy* that extensive research undeniably reveals "the surprisingly weak biological underpinnings of monogamy." They say that people's natural inclination is in fact to have sexual desire for multiple partners.

> Regardless of all that is out there questioning monogamy, a large majority of us are still struggling against nature to make it work, with a strong belief that it is the right thing to do.

Having multiple partners may be our natural sexual inclination, but humans have found many reasons to overpower nature for some worthwhile causes. So regardless of all that is out there questioning monogamy, a large majority of us are still struggling against nature to make it work, with a strong belief that it is the right thing to do. We may at times experience turmoil, confusion, and frustration in our relationship, as well as boredom and discontent. As a result, we may venture on journeys that take us far away. But often our journeys are within, and they bring us closer to home when we remember the joys, pleasures, and intimacies of sticking with just our mate, a mate that knows us oh so well.

As we seek to find sexual passion in our lives, there will always be temptations and urges. Infidelity is, and always has been, a hot topic. My friends and I are not immune to the frequent gossip of who is cheating and who is being cheated. We all know of marriages that have ended in divorce due to infidelity, and we all know people who have "worked it out" after an affair was uncovered. One can only wonder at the number of affairs that have never and will never be revealed, not even to the closest of friends.

As we seek to find healthy and productive ways to create more passion in our own long-term relationship, we can learn a lot from these alternative lifestyles and from those that chose to seek passion outside their relationship, sometimes lying and cheating to do so. These journeys of others may help us find our way and direct us down a more productive path for our own relationship. Let's consider the following:

CARLA'S QUEST

Despite her devotion to her profession, Carla had found time to date *a lot*. She felt she could have written a Midwestern version of *Sex and the City*. While all her friends were having babies, she had remained single and career oriented even into her forties. However, when Carla finally did get married three years ago, she was more than ready to settle down.

At first, married life was great. She and her husband enjoyed many evenings going out to dinner, having people over to their newly decorated home, and just hanging out together on the sofa. And when either she or her husband returned home from a business trip, they would rip each other's clothes off before they even reached the bedroom. However, even with the frequency of their travel schedules keeping them apart at times, Carla was noticing that normality and routine were creeping into their sex life. She knew she needed to put some extra effort into it to ward off her increasing boredom. Maybe she was just too used to the variety she had in her single life, or maybe she just had to accept that the passion eventually slips away in a long-term relationship.

One evening in bed, Carla asked her husband, John, to tell her a dirty story. John's story was about Carla with another man. He told it to her as if he were secretly watching from the closet. The story resulted in John and Carla having really heated sex that night. Later, John told Carla that the fantasy of seeing or hearing about her with another man really excited him. Carla was afraid to admit it, but it really excited her as well. She did not want to tell John how much she missed the excitement of first-time sex with new and different partners. Carla was cautious because she very much valued her marriage and did not want to risk hurting or even destroying it over sex.

After continually fueling their sexual encounters with talk of Carla with another man, John began suggesting that Carla really do it. She had plenty of opportunity on the road with the plethora of married men who frequently propositioned her. Carla had heard of other women who admitted that the occasional thrill of a sexual affair brought renewed passion to the marital bed. But

Carla was worried that it could nevertheless have a detrimental effect on their relationship. John would, no doubt, find the retelling exciting, but would he be threatened by it?

Carla considered what had happened recently to her friend Mary. Mary had called Carla about a fight she was having with her husband. He was convinced she was "up to no good." She had gone to visit her mother in another city and had spent some time with old college friends. Every time he had called she had been out, and several times she did not answer her cell phone. Mary felt as if he was constantly checking up on her and did not trust her. She had just wanted a break from all her responsibilities at home and had really enjoyed her time with old friends. Why couldn't her husband have just happily given her this break? What did he think she was doing, anyway?

Mary's husband finally confessed that he thought she had an affair. Mary had taken so much grief that she almost wished she had, but she had always been faithful and really did deserve her husband's trust. They fought viciously about this. However, after the heat of the initial fight, Mary's relationship actually started to improve. Apparently just thinking she was having an affair was motivational for her husband. He was suddenly much more attentive to her needs. He was noticing Mary's efforts, complimenting her and wooing her again. He was even working out and running with renewed zest.

Carla noted that Mary had not even slept with another man, and the imagined tryst had almost caused major problems in her relationship. She also reasoned, however, that if John did feel threatened by an encounter between her and another man, the consequences might not be detrimental but in fact beneficial in the long run. Perhaps John would be motivated in the same way that Mary's husband was. She facetiously thought John could benefit from a few sit-ups, and men in general could always afford to be a little more attentive. Plus, in this instance, John would know what she was doing; in fact he really wanted her to do it.

Carla and John discussed all of Carla's concerns. They both felt that their relationship was secure enough, and they both knew that the affair would just be about sex. Carla was confident that she could easily detach herself emotionally and keep the encounter in perspective. And John professed to feel the same way.

Carla discussed the idea with one of her close girlfriends as well. At first Lana agreed that the arrangement sounded as if it might work out just fine. She also thought it would be easy for Carla to find a willing male participant. Even Lana, a stay-at-home mom, was aware of the opportunities available to have an affair if one were so inclined. The bookstore, the gym, the grocery store, and even PTA meetings were all places of abundant opportunity. Carla told her friend that she was also familiar with numerous Web sites that catered to married women looking for a "date." That comment reminded Lana of an acquaintance who had met a lover on the Internet. Her name was Eve, and her indiscretions led to disastrous results.

Eve's case was one Carla especially needed to consider. Eve had an affair, and her husband found out. In his great fear of the marriage ending, he convinced her that it would excite him to "share" in the affair by seeing a videotape of the sex act. He was able to persuade her of this by showing a great deal of sexual excitement even just hearing about what she had done. With guilt overwhelming her, she finally, reluctantly agreed to do what he asked. However, once he viewed the video, the marriage was over. Actually seeing his wife in the throes of passion with another man was entirely different than hearing a "story" about it. His jealousy consumed him, and he could not look at his wife the same way again. All the marriage counseling in the world could not erase the permanent images in his mind of what she had done. Eve is now divorced and will tell us that unless we want our marriage to be over, we should not let our mate find out about an affair, or perhaps the best advice might be not to have one in the first place.

Lana questioned how anyone could be as foolish as Eve was. How could she in her right mind videotape the affair and show it to her husband? In actuality, she was not in her right mind. Eve wanted so much to reconnect with her spouse. Passionate love-making with her husband had suddenly returned once she had described for him the details of what she had done. His renewed excitement for her was what she had wanted all along. To feel sexy and desired again by her husband was a dream come true. And she agreed with him when he said he was entitled to the video. In this confused state of mind, Eve granted her husband's request, thinking it was the least she could do to make up for her indiscretions. Eve made a critical mistake.

When Lana was finished recounting what happened to Eve, Carla was really worried. John expressed such a strong desire to make his fantasy a reality and hear about her exploits with another man, but would that reality be something that he could live with? Maybe the fantasy would be better left as just that — a fantasy.

Carla also had a nagging concern that John was expressing a strong desire for her to do this simply because he thought it was what she really wanted. He was very perceptive and knew that she was feeling a little concerned about the monotony in their lovemaking. She absolutely did not want him to agree to this if it was really just for her. But how could she really know? Carla considered the fact that "you never *really* know" what someone is thinking.

Lana brought up another good point. Would Carla *really* be

comfortable sharing with John the intimate details of her sexual encounter? If the sex was great, how would that affect John's ego? Would comparison issues arise for either of them? (Lana suggested that, no matter what the reality was, Carla would have to tell John that her lover had a "small one.") Conversely, if it was a bad experience for Carla, John's fantasy of his wife with another man would be spoiled, and neither of them would have reaped any benefit at all from the encounter.

Carla was seeing too many potential pitfalls in making this fantasy a reality. She was no longer sure that she or John could really look at the experience as just a physical occurrence, without any meaning *and* without any comparisons that could lead to insecurity in the marriage. This journey seemed to be too perilous. But the fantasy was taking on a life of its own. The question was, where should they go with it next? Did Carla really want to cross this line that might be hard to cross back from?

We will find out what Carla decided in chapter 7. For now, it would be helpful to look at the line Jessie *did* cross.

JESSIE'S QUEST

Jessie had just received a promotion and was taking a few days off before the executive retreat she was to attend over the weekend. The children were still at school, and Jessie was alone in the house. She was rummaging through the back of her husband's closet, looking for the black carry-on bag. It was then that she saw the milk crate. It appeared to be full of *National Geographic* magazines, but a DVD that was sticking up caught her eye. When she looked closer she realized the crate was actually full of *Playboy* and *Penthouse* magazines, and a few movies that, from the titles, Jessie was sure were pornographic. She was enraged.

Jessie and her husband, Rob, had been through this before. Jessie felt that it was not only inappropriate to have such materials in the house because of the children but that the items were degrading to women and just plain sick. Apparently Rob was ignoring all of her concerns. He had for a long time complained about their sex life. Often the jabs were disguised as humorous banter, but sometimes his dissatisfaction came out in full force, especially when they were fighting about something.

As Jessie thought about the situation, she realized Rob's complaints were not as frequent anymore. Maybe he had finally accepted that in a long-term relationship the passion would necessarily slip away. Jessie had told him on a number of occasions how unreasonable he was being to expect them to still make passionate love after twelve years of marriage and two children. Plus, she worked so hard at her career, and the children needed her. She did not have the time or the energy to "play sex" with her husband. He needed to grow up and accept the reality of adulthood.

Jessie had trouble getting the milk crate out of her mind. Why was her husband so obsessed with sex? She recognized that he wanted sex more than she did, but it was not as if she never "did it" with him. She would sometimes even pretend to enjoy herself — whatever it took to get the experience over with as soon as possible so that she could get to sleep. She always had a busy day coming up and really needed her rest.

The next day, Jessie found herself drawn back to the milk crate, and she leafed through the magazines inside. Had anything been touched? She looked at the photos and tried to imagine what he was doing with this stuff. She had never thought of herself as very sexual but rather somewhat inhibited. Jessie had been raised to believe that it was somehow unclean to have sexual thoughts. The photo in front of Jessie was of a very beautiful, voluptuous blonde with a naked muscular man standing behind her. He was holding the woman's full, round breasts. Jessie thought of her husband looking at the photo and touching himself. It did not dawn on her that she was getting aroused. She quickly and angrily threw the magazine back into the crate and shoved the image out of her mind.

That night Jessie could not sleep, and she went downstairs and saw a light on in the den. She heard Rob typing at the computer. Assuming he was working, she tiptoed past the den on her way to the kitchen, and as she did, she heard the distinct ping of an instant message coming in. Then she heard Rob make a soft sigh and start typing again. What was he doing? Who was he chatting with at this hour? Jessie pushed the door open, and there was Rob, sitting at the computer with his pants down and obviously very aroused. The computer blurted "good-bye" as Rob immediately closed the window on the computer screen, and that broke the silent, shocked stare between them.

Jessie lost it. Finding pornography in their home and now seeing him so obviously having cybersex were too much. She asked her husband why he was so obsessed with sex. Rob responded by questioning why she was such a cold fish. Jessie was never there for him — her attentions went to everyone else, and there was nothing left for her husband. Her going through the motions with him in bed was no fun anymore. She was never interested in trying anything new or different. She had said it herself — she could live without it. But he could not, so what did she expect him to do? Rob pointed out that at least he was not having an affair. She should be thankful that cybersex was all he was doing without her.

The next day, as Jessie boarded the plane for her retreat, she thought about her sex life. Maybe there was something wrong with her. Why did she care so little about sex? After the children, sex seemed to become frivolous. It had not always been that way, though. She tried to call up in her mind the details of those early sexual encounters with her husband. He had been so patient with her, always ensuring that she reached climax before he reached his own. In the few times she had (sinfully, she thought) gone all the way with boyfriends in college, not one of them had ever taken the time to satisfy her, and she had never felt comfortable asking for what she wanted. Until Rob, she was sure it was her own fault that she had not climaxed, and she would fake it so her boyfriend would not know the truth.

Jessie was still very angry with Rob. He was so demanding, and he had managed to turn the whole sex issue into something that was her fault. She had enough demands and pressures on her as it was. She felt she was never there for the kids as much as she should be, and now, with this promotion, she would be even busier at work. Why did Rob not see that his demands were so unfair to her?

He had said she was not fun anymore. She could be fun — lots of fun. The gang at work thought she was a fun boss. She could banter and even cleverly respond to a sexual innuendo when one was tossed her way. And although she rarely paid attention, she knew men still looked at her. Jessie thought she could even be sexy if she wanted to.

As Jessie got off the plane and walked through the airport terminal, she began to pay attention. She looked into people's eyes and even smiled at a few attractive men rushing by her. There was nothing wrong with her . . . was there?

The executive retreat was supposed to act as a morale booster and as a thank-you to the sales team. Jessie's department had planned the event and hired the speakers. One speaker in particular captured Jessie's attention, and she found herself tuning in to him. He was a motivational speaker, and he was talking about creating a "passion" for the corporate goal. He told the executives to turn inward and find the passion within themselves, then to take it to a higher level and go for the gold. "We all have it in us; we just have to let it out." This was the canned motivational crap that Jessie had heard a million times, but she was not thinking about sales goals — she was thinking about sex.

That night she met the senior vice president of sales for drinks before they were to take the group out to dinner. He was new to the company and was trying hard to establish himself with her. Her first impression was that he was the typical salesman, rather arrogant and a little too friendly. Tonight, though, he seemed different. He was very relaxed and quickly put her at ease as well. Some members of the sales group stopped in at the bar and asked if they could skip dinner and head straight to a club they wanted to check out. He sent them on their way, and suddenly Jessie was alone with him for dinner.

Jessie had not felt this alive in a long time. She even thought that maybe he was flirting with her. After the nasty fight with her husband, Jessie felt entitled to enjoy herself. She was obviously not a cold fish; this man did not think so, anyway. He appeared to find her exciting and interesting. The conversation was very stimulating and it flowed easily. The cocktails, and now the wine with dinner, made Jessie feel warm and sexy. She was now flirting shamelessly, and she blushed at her own boldness.

Jessie was enthralled with everything about this man, especially his voice. She melted with the warmth of it. When he spoke softly to her, Jessie lost all ability to think straight, to focus. His voice was carrying her to a place that was still and peaceful, but at the same time it was stirring passions within her that had too long been quiet.

Jessie was not thinking about what was happening. She blindly let him lead her to his hotel room. She wanted him to desire her the way those women in the porn magazines were desired. He said all the right things. He made her feel as if she were the hottest, sexiest woman alive. She had never felt like this before. He was so practiced and so talented — she was swept away by his touch.

Jessie had the best sex of her life that night. She had never known it could be like that. What was it about this man? She wanted to know. The rest of the retreat, Jessie spent every minute she could with him. He was dynamic and energetic, and he made her feel that she was too. Her senses had come alive, and she was overwhelmed.

Jessie was struggling with the reality of what was happening between her and this man. How much of it was timing, due in large part to the problems she was having in her marriage, and how much was truly a soulful connection? She wanted to believe the latter, for she was encountering a rush of new emotions and a great deal of reflection as a result of the experience. Whatever the reason, Jessie chose to look at the encounter as a gift, a gift she stole for herself, a gift she deserved, a gift she very much enjoyed opening . . . a gift she wanted to keep.

As she boarded the plane to head home, Jessie knew the experience would not end there. In her mind, he was now the fantasy — everything her husband was not. Although they worked out of offices in different cities, she would see her lover again. She could not stop thinking about him and what they had experienced together. Jessie was sure it was not "just sex" for either of them. She was sure she was not confusing great sex with something more meaningful. Her mind was consumed with all the passionate thoughts that had so long been suppressed. Surely she could not feel this alive and this inspired if the encounter had not meant anything to him.

Things were very bad at Jessie's house. The relationship was severely strained before she had left for her business trip. Now the situation was worse. Jessie was experiencing a wide range of emotions. She felt very hostile toward her husband, guilty about what she had done, excited about her newly found passion, obsessed with thoughts of her lover, and completely unsure of what to do about it all. For someone who just a week prior did not even have time for sex and thought she had accepted the loss of sexual passion, this was new territory. It was amazing how much energy she was suddenly finding to put into just *thinking* about sex.

Jessie's guilt was so overwhelming that she was actually blaming her husband for what she had done. It was his fault that she had been feeling something was sexually wrong with her. She had been left with no choice but to prove him wrong. Besides, he was cheating on her anyway, maybe not physically but certainly emotionally with his online affair, and it was obvious where that was heading.

Still, Jessie really had to work to justify what she had done. She knew in her heart how hurtful this affair would be to Rob. She knew how upset she was that he was just having cybersex. How did she get to this place where she was now thinking of cybersex as "*just* cybersex"? She had to quickly push that thought out of her mind. It was far too devastating to think about all this . . . her secret, her lie, and her knowledge that she had failed to keep her vows.

Jessie's confusion was greatly amplified by the newly found passion within her. Had these sexual feelings been dormant all these years? Suddenly sex was all she could think about. She conjured up images of the affair and masturbated a lot. She tried to remember when she had ever felt such a sexual rush about someone. She could not recall, even early on in her relationship with her husband, ever feeling this much intensity just being naked with a man. And she certainly had never wanted to be with someone enough to be deceitful about it.

Jessie wanted to know more. She had little sexual experience before marriage and had not experimented at all with her husband. Now she wanted to try it all. She felt that in the secret world of her affair, she could be that naughty girl she never imagined she could be. She could go for what she wanted. She could even *ask* for it.

Her lover said all the right things. And Jessie believed that something that felt this right could not possibly be wrong. In her mind, he was everything she had ever dreamed of but doubted really existed. Fantasy and reality had become one. He was the romance-novel hero, the man she could not refuse. Even though she knew relatively little about him, her judgment was so blurred by the discovery of great sex that she believed this lover must be her "once in a lifetime" love. She started plotting ways she could be with him — permanently. But was this man truly a "once in a lifetime" love or merely an inspirational pawn in the natural progression of her sexual awakening?

Some might ask, how could an intelligent, successful career woman such as Jessie so easily mistake great sex for love? Could she possibly be so naive? Unfortunately it is easier to confuse the two than one would think. The emotional intimacy of the act of sex itself was blurring Jessie's vision of the path she was on. Jessie was undergoing a sexual awakening, a journey of sorts toward a sexual renewal in her life. Whether this sexual awakening was due to meeting the "right" person, or whether it was just the right time in Jessie's life, was something that she needed to figure out.

Jessie turned to her close friend for counsel. Her confidante pointed out to her that the vast majority of men willing to have an affair with a married woman are primarily interested because, as a married woman, she is *not* available. This man knew Jessie belonged to someone else, that she was married with children. Going into the affair, her lover probably felt that the risk of emotional entanglement and complications was decreased dramatically. Did Jessie really think that he had any intention of maintaining a long-term relationship with her? How much of what she was feeling toward him was created in her own mind, and how much of it was he really reciprocating? Jessie was opening herself up to the likelihood of rejection and emotional pain, whether she ended the affair or he did. Jessie's friend noted that, either way, it would end. It *always* did.

Even if her lover wanted more, Jessie knew she had to think about her children. Her kids, of course, were much more important than anything else. How could she turn their world upside down in her pursuit of passion? Even if she was supposed to be with this man, she was already committed to someone else, and the children needed that commitment to remain intact.

So how was Jessie going to find the strength to emotionally detach? She was experiencing major comparison repercussions. She felt her lover was so much more sexually satisfying than Rob had ever been. How could she go back to what now seemed so mediocre and be happy with it? Jessie's close friend reminded her that the affair was new and told her that first-time sex is always more passionate and more exciting. But Jessie kept thinking, how could she happily go back to the overly familiar now that she had been exposed to the excitement of discovering something new and different?

Jessie would have to be able to take what she learned from the experience and somehow find a way to use it positively in her marital bedroom. This would be a tall order. Would Jessie ever be able to detach and put the affair properly into perspective? Or would it destroy her marriage? We will see where her perilous journey takes her in the next chapter.

PERILOUS *AND* FATEFUL

One woman told me, "For so many years, I had been knee-deep in raising my family. To be romanced and pursued again was something I thought was lost to me now that I have been married for nearly twenty years. But here I was with another man, sipping wine, holding hands, feeling beautiful and alive again." Another woman confided, "My affair was like those office scenes in a porno movie my husband would put in the DVD player — just so spontaneous and hot. It had been a long, long time since I felt that kind of heat. His desire was such an ego boost."

So many of us in our thirties, forties, or beyond just want to feel young, sexy, and desired again. According to the U.S. Bureau of Labor Statistics, about 60 percent of women are in the workplace. The rest of us are at soccer practice, the gym, the club, PTA meetings, charity functions, etc. We are meeting people, including men. These men often see us in something other than sweatpants, with makeup on *and* showing our best behavior. The opportunities to have an affair are endless. Why do some women take this perilous journey? Is it a solution to the loss of passion at home? Or is it a wake-up call foreshadowing the finale?

One woman I met on a volunteer project told me about an affair she once had with her boss. She admitted, "Work for me had become so consuming. It was like a separate life for me, separate and apart from my family life. I spent so much time with my boss. He really appreciated all the time and effort I put into the company. He was there. We were both lonely for attention. It just happened." Another woman said of her affair, "It was exciting. I felt so young, sexy, and desirable again. In my late thirties, after two kids and lots of, well, life behind me, it was really nice to feel like there was a lot more to come. My sexual excitement was like I never remembered it . . . out of this world. My skin felt on fire and I was frantic. I could not believe it could be this hot."

From these comments and from other conversations I have had with many women both in person and on the Internet, I have compiled the following Passion Seekers' list of why women are choosing to take the path to infidelity.

Why Some Women Take Perilous Journeys

- They want to be wooed and get that "date treatment" again.
- They wish to feel sexy and desired.
- They need a wake-up call for themselves and their spouse, renewing the effort to be attentive.
- The affair gives them a secret source of strength.
- The tryst provides the incentive to leave their husband.
- They are seeking that which is lacking in their marriage/relationship.
- They want to get even with their mate for cheating or for other perceived wrongs.
- They want excitement and adventure in an otherwise boring existence.
- They are thrilled by having a secret and the risk of being caught.
- They want to feel the passion again, including the newness and excitement. (Not being able to see each other without great effort often keeps the affair passionate.)

- The affair just happens — they are out in the world, meeting new people, traveling, and having more opportunities presented to them.

After listening to the stories of so many women who have cheated on their mate for one reason or another, I have uncovered some universal truths about the current state of "affairs." First, it would seem that one of the only *real* advantages to having an affair would be the possibility of being wooed and desired, and experiencing momentary sexual pleasure different from the routine. The excitement of first-time sex is a big draw. There is, of course, no guarantee that the experience will be a pleasurable one, and memories can be hard to erase. The question we must ask ourselves is whether the momentary thrill of the affair is worth all the risks involved, including damaging or losing the long-term relationship with our spouse, whose feelings we presumably care about.

Second, the vast majority of affairs are kept and *must be kept* secret from the spouse. Most realize that acting on the desire to be with someone else would be hurtful to their spouse, and therefore they vigorously work to keep it a secret. As with Jessie, one would then have to live with the secret, the lie, and the guilt that one's vows were not kept. Nothing was solved. It was like that piece of rich chocolate dessert — something that was enjoyable and gave her a moment of pleasure. Now, like the chocolate that will go to her hips, the experience will forever be with her unless she puts a great deal of effort into working it out of her system.

Add to this the question of whether a woman involved in an affair is even able to take the experience for what it is — just sex. Jessie is the perfect example of how emotional detachment is not always as easy as some of our male counterparts make it sound. Sure, this sort of detachment is simple if the attraction is purely a physical one and remains so. For many women, however, sex is not what the affair is really all about. For some, getting to know their lover is part of the game, and as a result they risk liking the person as well as wanting to make love to him. As Jessie found out, great (or even just good) sex can often feel as if it is more than *just sex*.

Keeping the various thoughts and emotions compartmentalized in the here and now is not an easy task, especially for those struggling with marital discontent (which is probably the reason for the affair to begin with). Our youthful romantic image of the ideal lover or elusive soul mate can enter our mind, and the fantasy can take over. Suddenly this new and exciting lover may consume our psyche, and reality may take a vacation. This experience has been covered in literature ad nauseam. The reality, however, is never happily ever after.

Our discussion has not even begun to touch on the moral and religious issues involved in having an affair. The depth that those issues require is beyond the scope and purpose of this book but must be considered when contemplating an extramarital affair. Also, from a practical health standpoint, we must always consider the risk of exposure to sexually transmitted diseases. Physical pleasure is never worth taking unnecessary risks with one's health and certainly not with the health of one's spouse as well.

The bottom line is that an affair is *not* going to solve anything, least of all boredom in the bedroom at home. Only we, together with our spouse, can do that. The solution is not to seek outside of our relationship that which is missing in it, but rather to work toward creating passion with our spouse. An affair may bring us momentary pleasure and perceived intimacy, but then we have to go home to reality, to exactly what was there before. So, instead of having an affair, we should try a new approach with our old lover. At the very least we will have fun trying, and with some effort and creativity, sex might just end up feeling new again.

CHAPTER SIX

THE JOURNEY HOME

REDISCOVERING THE PASSION *WITHIN US*

WEATHERING THE QUEST FOR PASSION

We return now to Jessie's perilous journey. In the following pages, we will see how Jessie's recollections of an early sexual encounter that went horribly awry will reveal to us the emotional impact youthful "mistakes" can have on our present-day intimate relationships. Recognizing the influence of her traumatic past experience, Jessie takes a journey of self-discovery. She acknowledges for the first time her innate primal urges and needs.

We can learn from Jessie not only about the perils of infidelity but about how all of us can take a journey of sorts *within*. The end of Jessie's journey and the new beginnings in her life reveal examples of how each of us can create a renewed sexual self. All of the experiences in this chapter expose the importance of "owning the problem" and utilizing the power within to take the lead and initiate change.

Jessie's Perilous Journey

Without even realizing it, Jessie had set out on a journey and was now very far from home. She was not sure how to return or even if she wanted to return. Jessie now knew that the fantasy really existed — earth-shattering passion and mind-blowing sex. To make matters worse, in an effort to justify her indiscretions, Jessie was crediting her lover as the source of all her newfound sexual passion and desire, and rashly elevating him to the status of elusive soul mate.

Her mind did not allow her to recall the sparks ever having been like this with her husband or with any man, even when the relationship was new. Although Jessie did not really know her lover, she refused to accept that her sudden desire had nothing to do with him at all. She was ignoring the real journey she was on. Jessie wanted to believe that her new feelings were all caused by this man and that he was just *so right* for her. There was no denying how he possessed her mind. He was adventurous and intelligent. He was sexy and mysterious. He was the fantasy.

Jessie was seeing signs in everything, believing that this affair was so much more, that he really was "the one." It was a sign that they had both recently experienced the accidental death of a friend. It was a sign that as a child he had completed a school project on her hometown, even though he grew up thousands of miles away. To Jessie, these "signs" were not mere coincidences. She placed significance on them to justify to herself that this was not just a tawdry affair but rather a fated match.

She was trying to live the storybook fantasy, ignoring the fact that the Madame Bovarys and Anna Kareninas of the world do *not* live happily ever after. Jessie worked at tricking her mind into believing that the affair was not all about sex but rather a truly soulful connection. She was so inspired that she had to perform mental gymnastics in an attempt to downplay the events in her mind and function in her everyday roles and responsibilities.

Jessie's dilemma was clearly a case of glamorized romance with a man she had idealized in her mind. Although she did not really know him, he remained, in her thoughts, perfect. At this point, Jessie was not allowing herself to recognize that her feelings were in sharp contrast to the reality of true love — love that comes from acceptance and knowing someone inside and out. This kind of love may not always be new and exciting, but it is safe, real, and meaningful.

Even as time passed and her home life continued with a facade of normalcy, she could not get her lover out of her mind. The journey within was proving to be arduous and even painful. She recognized that she was unable to determine what was real. Only her children kept her from falling off the edge and into the great unknown.

Very quickly, her lover's passionate expressions became few and far between. She was the one who usually initiated contact. He would always respond, but he never e-mailed or phoned on his own. She rationalized this in her mind. Her lover was being considerate and cautious so that her husband would not find out, but in lucid moments she knew she was making excuses for him.

A day or so would go by, and Jessie would not think of him. She worked very hard and kept very busy to keep her mind from wandering back down that path. The hardest moments were at night, as she closed her eyes to sleep. Jessie would see him in her mind and start plotting ways to make fantasy a reality.

As the days turned to weeks and the weeks turned to months, Jessie could not entirely tune out the sane voice of reality within her. When she tried to look at the problem objectively, she realized that her lover was not giving himself to her on any emotional level and was making little effort to get to know her. He never asked what she was doing or how things were going. It was Jessie who was making all the intimate gestures. In reality, he had very little interest in talking at all — genuine intimacy did not appear to be on his agenda.

As he slowly distanced himself with longer periods of time before responding to e-mails and phone calls, Jessie drifted back down to earth. Her mind had played many tricks on her. She eventually discovered that writing everything down was very beneficial. In doing so Jessie was beginning to see the affair for the fantasy that it was, and she started to put the experience properly into perspective. Was it really all an illusion that she had created in her mind? Jessie *logically* knew all along that the fantasy could never really be a permanent reality but nevertheless allowed herself to believe that it could. What was she really trying to grasp on to? She knew that he was not really the perfect image she had built up in her mind and that she was not being real either.

Coming back home was the right thing to do. The children needed their parents to stay together. With her kids foremost in her mind, Jessie slowly and painfully traveled back to reality. Her baggage was much heavier for the return, filled now with so many passionate memories, although much of them figments of her own imagination.

Would she ever be able to find her way home again entirely? A part of Jessie was still out there on that journey, needing to take the affair farther into the vast unknown. She did not know if she could ever go back to the ordinary, the familiar, and the mediocre. She liked that passionate person she became with her lover, or at least she liked the fantasy in her mind — maybe that was what she was trying so hard to hold on to.

Jessie was tortured by the need to let go of her lover *but at the same time not let go of the passionate person she had found within herself.* So Jessie had to struggle to redirect her desire, her newfound needs. Forever changed, she realized that to return from this journey required that she find a way to keep the passion alive within herself, without her lover there — literally or figuratively.

Jessie was becoming disgusted with herself. The guilt and internal anguish were the punishments she felt she rightly deserved for the sinful betrayal she had committed. She fought the condemning voices inside her, determined to learn from all this and somehow forgive herself. If her marriage was to survive and be healthy again, the affair had to be taken for what it was (and what it could only have been) — a physically pleasurable release. Jessie now needed to turn inward and address the real issues.

Jessie said good-bye to her lover. She felt foolish; she realized now how very practiced he had been and how good at getting what he wanted. The blame, though, was not really his. Jessie had briefly lost her rationality through no one's fault but her own. Realizing this, she could now appreciate her affair for what it was and hopefully find her way back home.

Jessie owed her husband an opportunity to venture out on a passion quest with her. First, she had to come home and be completely at ease with herself. Then, and only then, could she and her husband enjoy a journey within the confines of their marital vows. Jessie would undoubtedly find it much harder to set out again, because she was now weary from the emotional burden of the perilous journey she had already undertaken.

Internal Explorations

What is important to realize about infidelity is that there are few women who successfully manage to keep their emotions out of their sexual encounters. Most would agree that *making love is an emotional event*. Thus, an affair rarely ends up being just about sex: an emotional entanglement — sometimes one-sided, sometimes not — is bound to occur.

Jessie is the perfect example of this kind of emotional confusion. She lost herself in the fantasy of a new passionate encounter. When she came crashing back down to earth, she felt foolish, guilty, and ashamed. Jessie had wanted to feel sexy again and to understand what all the fuss surrounding sex was about, but mostly she was angry with her husband and wished to be someone other than the "cold fish" she saw reflected in his eyes.

Jessie can never change what she did. She can never erase the painful journey she undertook. But she was eventually able to recognize what the affair was really about. Jessie kept a journal and confided in her closest friend. In doing so, she began a long and painful path toward self-discovery. Her perilous journey was really just the beginning of a far more meaningful one — that of discovering and awakening the passion within.

A Journey into the Past

While writing in her journal in an effort to put the affair into proper perspective, Jessie was recognizing for the first time how her upbringing and her earliest sexual encounters continued to

impact her present-day intimate sexual relationship and ultimately her whole concept as a sexual being.

Jessie revealed in her writings that when she was growing up,
sex was a taboo topic in her house. "Relations" were between a
husband and wife, and were for the purpose of procreating —
that is what her religious education taught her about sex, and
that was basically the extent of her knowledge on the subject.
Jessie's real education came the hard way not long after she left
home for college.

At school, Jessie made friends and started going out to parties on weekends. Soon she noticed a fraternity guy named Mike.
They talked and flirted on several occasions, and one evening he
stopped by her dorm room. Things got a little heated. Jessie
reached a point where she was not comfortable and finally asked
Mike to leave. So far, the story is pretty typical. However, what
happened next was not.

A short while after her heartthrob left, there was a knock at
her door. When Jessie opened it, one of Mike's friends pushed
his way into her dorm room and shut the door. To Jessie's shock,
he started forcing himself on her and claimed that Mike had
said she would not mind. Jessie was stunned. She struggled and
pushed at him. Finally, he gave up and left the room, but the
nightmare was not over yet. Soon, another of Mike's friends
knocked at the door. This time Jessie refused to open it. He continued to bang on the door and bellow that he knew she "wanted
it." Jessie was mortified. Crying and shaking, she called her
dorm floor monitor, but no one answered the phone. Everyone
seemed to be out this night: the floor was quiet, too quiet, except
for the banging and yelling at her door.

For what seemed like an eternity, Jessie cried while the constant clamor outside her room continued. Finally, silence took

over, and Jessie's sobs slowly subsided. She lay curled in a ball on her bed, wishing she could make herself so small that she would disappear forever.

Unfortunately the experience was still not over. Jessie endured jeers and lewd sound effects whenever one of Mike's fraternity brothers passed her on campus. Her reputation suffered. She could not understand why this was happening to her, and she cursed herself for having ever let Mike into her dorm room. Why had she trusted him? She had made out with boys before, but never had she paid such a dear price for not "going all the way."

Jessie was very upset and sought help from the campus counseling office. The counselor listened to what Jessie described and stated that there was always an element of truth to rumors — what had Jessie done to encourage the young men to behave this way? Jessie was as hurt by this as she was by the horrid experience itself.

When I ask women to tell me about their early sexual encounters, many stories emerge that are often unpleasant. We all have something in our sexual past that has shaped who we are today and how we feel about sex and intimacy. But how do these early encounters and pressures from the opposite sex impact a woman's long-term ability to trust her own sexuality, not to mention her motivation to feed her sexual and passionate self? Certainly, in Jessie's case, she carried baggage on her passion journey — baggage that caused her to mistrust not only the sexual feelings of others but her own as well. For many years, a combination of her rigid upbringing and her early experience in college caused Jessie to suppress her sexuality and believe that sex was trouble with a capital "T."

INSTINCT, NEED, AND ATTITUDE

Jessie's story teaches us to recognize the impact of our past experiences on how we think about sex and sexual relationships. In the process of such self-examination, we will perhaps locate, stay in touch with, or rediscover our basic sexual needs and instincts. We can then be better prepared to adjust our attitude and cultivate our sexual creativity to expose the passion within.

> We must feed our sexual needs just as we feed our nutritional ones.

After the incident in college, Jessie waited a long time before ever trusting a man enough to be intimate with him. She was sure that if she gave in to passionate feelings, she would pay a heavy price. The few times that she did have sex before her husband was in the picture, Jessie was not able to let go or relax enough to have her own sexual needs met or even to ask for what she wanted. She had given in only because of a strong sense of obligation to her boyfriend. He seemed to need it so bad. Sex was really important to him, and she did not want to lose him as a boyfriend. Unfortunately, in not knowing how to ask for what she needed to enjoy the experience, Jessie did not even realize what she was missing — passion, not to mention orgasm, eluded her.

Jessie's years of suppression finally ended when she had the affair. She acknowledged for the first time her innate urges and needs. She discovered that the act of sex itself was not an obligation but a real source of incredible pleasure and ultimate intimacy. Jessie began to appreciate sex as a gift to herself. She was not making love out of a sense of obligation to anyone. In sharing her story, Jessie reminds us all that sexual relations with our mate are a passionate gift of love. We must never view sex as an *obligation.*

We must feed our sexual needs just as we feed our nutritional ones. This is what Jessie learned the hard way. We must remind ourselves that sex is as instinctual and primitive as our need for food and water. If we stop fighting (or ignoring) the forces of nature and instead embrace them, we will come a long way toward embracing our passionate selves.

We must learn to love, *really love,* sex again.

Just as it was for Jessie before her affair, our own daily grind and outside pressures of children and work often force our sexual needs to the back burner. We sometimes consciously deny that they even exist. But the fact remains that a healthy level of passion in our life goes a long way toward sexual satisfaction and fulfillment, and ultimately toward the intimate and long-term relationship we crave with our mate.

We are obligated to feed this basic need and recognize its existence inside each of us. To deny ourselves is to starve our very core. We become like an anorexic: we starve our body of its basic nutritional needs because in our mind we do not need food. We have to work very hard to overcome our disease and retrain our mind about food. The anorexic needs to learn to love eating again. Although we are not risking death by not having sex, we are risking the death of passion in our lives and the loss of intimacy that goes with it. So we must learn to love, *really love,* sex again. We must accept this basic human need, make it an important part of our everyday lives, and properly feed it. If we do so, our intimate relationship will *passionately* improve.

Finding the Way Back Home

Without even realizing it at the time, Jessie had been seeking a solution to her stagnant and unfulfilling sexual relationship with her husband. She came to understand that she had journeyed down the wrong path. She decided her solution was not to travel outside her marriage but rather to find the path that led home. For the first time, Jessie was recognizing that the problem was not so much what was missing in her relationship with her husband but rather what was missing in *her*.

Jessie had ignored her own innate sexual needs. She had denied the instinctual urges. She had focused all her energy on her children and her career and everything but her intimate relationship with her mate. The sudden and extreme journey she undertook with her affair forced Jessie to learn the hard way. She had unknowingly taken an emotional plunge into discovering her sexuality, and gravely risked her marriage in the process.

The affair began for Jessie as an effort to validate herself and her sexuality — to feel sexy. She had unknowingly sought out that which was missing in her relationship and, most important, in herself. She was angry with her husband, but deep down she realized he had a point. Their marriage was no longer stimulating, only safe and secure. Her cry-for-help actions of allowing the affair to happen did not solve anything and instead risked the marriage itself. Jessie eventually realized that the solution for her was certainly not to seek a new relationship or a rescuer. Only she could rescue herself and, ultimately, the relationship as well.

While having the affair, Jessie had discovered a passionate self. She became determined to redirect that energy and passion into her marriage. This could begin only with a *permanent* adjustment in her attitude — her attitude toward herself and her sexuality, and finally her attitude toward her sexual relationship with her husband.

GETTING THERE — A RENEWED SEXUAL SELF

Attitude! Attitude! Attitude!

To succeed on the journey, some may need a major attitude overhaul. They, like Jessie, will have to redirect newfound passions and open up to what is right there in front of them. Others may simply need to put more effort into making love or place a higher priority on their sexual relationship with their mate. A good example is the story of my friend Claire.

One day, in tears, Claire revealed to me that she thought her husband was having an affair. I encouraged her to fight fire with fire . . . if she really wanted to hold it together. Where was that fighting nature of hers? I knew her when we were in college. She was a go-getter with both her schoolwork and her love life. Claire always went after (and usually got) the most sought-after guys. I reminded her about her attitude in college. She got the best because she felt entitled to the best and expected the best. She needed to dig deep and bring that confident attitude back to the surface.

Claire was entitled to a lot better than she was receiving from her husband, but she no longer acted entitled. She did not realize it, but she was getting out of her relationship exactly what she was putting into it — next to nothing. If she wanted to redirect her husband's passions back toward her, she needed to re-create that attitude that demanded attention. She had the power within her — I had seen it before. There was a time when Claire believed she was sexy, and therefore she was. That sexy attitude was a frame of mind she carried with her everywhere she went. Even though she did not feel that way now, I had complete confidence that she could rediscover that attitude.

I suggested that, if necessary, she start by faking a sexy attitude. I knew that before long she would not be faking anymore — the attitude would again take over and empower her. Soon, she would not be acting — and he would take notice. She could not control his behavior or his attitude toward the relationship, but she could control *her own* attitude and behavior. She could choose to take better care of herself. If she felt a new outfit or a makeover would help, she could do that. She could choose to believe she was sexy and desirable. She could choose to act as if she was. Before too long, he would notice the change, and if the marriage meant anything to him, he would positively respond. And if the marriage meant nothing to him, at least she would be able to exit with her head held high, knowing she had not just passively let the relationship slip away.

The research I have conducted and the stories I have collected all reveal one common theme: if we are looking to dramatically improve our sexual relationship with our mate, we must build a passionate frame of mind. For now, we will forget the technique books, the sex seminars, the lingerie, and the sex toys. Instead we will focus on our attitude toward sex and passion. Passionate sex is a state of mind where the only tools needed are a positive attitude and a little creativity and enthusiasm.

The ultimate goal is to put ourselves in a sexy frame of mind and help create a passionate mood. How we accomplish this begins with our attitude. Women are built to be sexy. We are all sexy, and we have to believe it and use it! We may say we do not *feel* sexy, but that is just the point — our sexual attitude is *all* about what we are feeling. If we feel sexy, we become sexy. Our mind is the sexiest tool of all. We must believe we have what it takes. Confidence is sexy!

> Passionate sex is a state of mind where the only tools needed are a positive attitude and a little creativity and enthusiasm.

Remember, the secret weapon of every sexy woman is her mind. Our attitude is what makes us feel sexy. Sure, we all know how our body image affects our attitude, and we find it hard to feel sexy when we focus on our "flaws." We must instead play up our positives and focus our time and energy on what gives us that sexy feeling. We do not need to make this complicated. This could be something as simple as a new pair of shoes, a push-up bra, a good workout in the gym, or a spa treatment. This is not about him — this is for us.

Taking it one step further, at Passion Seekers' parties we make a list of what makes us feel sexy and what makes us sexually excited. Each list is unique. We then give ourselves permission to seek out new sensations. Maybe something on our friend's list is something we never tried or thought of — maybe it will inspire us to seek out what we need to do for ourselves to take hold of that sexy feeling and attitude. For example, here are some of the answers I received when I asked Passion Seekers to tell me what gets them *hot:*

Some Wild Ways Passion Seekers Get Excited

- Having ear sucked on for a few minutes
- Receiving a foot rub
- Completing about twenty to twenty-five abdominal exercises on the Roman Chair
- Leaning on a vibrating washing machine during the spin cycle
- Feeling the spray of a pulsating showerhead

- Sunbathing topless
- Doing sit-ups and Kegels to increase the blood flow before sex
- Having nipples sucked on
- Watching people have sex

We can find a way to be alone with our mate for the night, take a hot shower, slip on something sexy, put on some mood music, drink a glass of wine, light some candles, and read a sexy story, then invite our mate to bed. The sexy attitude is there, buried under the pile of to-dos. We will put aside the grocery list and not think of the laundry, the car pools, or the job assignment. Instead, we will remember his sensual touch, his breath on our neck, and the fun of turning him on and thrill of making him want us.

Discovering and Awakening the Passion Within

Jessie's attitude toward making love with her husband had always been one of obligation. And her attitude toward the act of sex itself was worse. She had been inattentive to Rob's needs, and her own, all these years. She always felt she had no energy left to enjoy sex, let alone pay much attention to Rob's sexual needs *or* even recognize her own. Jessie realized that if she was more attentive to her sexual relationship with her mate — instead of treating her husband's desires as if they were immature obsessions — things would improve in her marriage.

Jessie's divorced friend Beth told her about the great sexual divide in her marriage that had played a large role in ending the relationship. She described her sexual incapability with her husband as a constant power struggle between his needs and hers. Beth was full of regrets. She had constantly told herself that she was too tired or too busy to put any effort into making love. Beth felt that if she had only looked forward to those intimate encounters and shown a little enthusiasm for them rather than viewing sex with her mate as a chore, maybe their relationship would not have fallen apart.

Whether out of fear of her marriage ending, guilt over the affair, or a newly inflamed sexual passion, Jessie enthusiastically made love to her husband that night. It was the beginning of a new attitude for Jessie regarding her sexual relationship with her mate.

Jessie planned a tropical vacation alone with her husband. Rob was thrilled to have her all to himself for the first time in years. The atmosphere at the resort was romantic and sensual. It was the start of a new journey for Jessie — one that she and her mate would take together.

"Sensational" New Beginnings

The warmth of the sun only intensified Jessie's sensations as she lay close to her husband on the beach. With her eyes closed, she felt him rubbing the suntan oil onto her. When Jessie opened her eyes again, he was no longer beside her. She quickly scanned the sunbathing crowd and spotted him near the outdoor bar with a drink in his hand. He was conversing with other resort guests, so relaxed and confident. Jessie noticed no one but him. Her husband was tall, tan, and built in just the way she liked. As she watched him, the bright sunshine seemed to slip away and clouds moved in. The welcome relief from the heat soothed her tanned skin, and the wind provided a gentle massage. Jessie closed her eyes as the first raindrops fell on her near-naked body. She felt each one as a welcome tender touch.

Slowly, bathers around her rose and gathered their belongings, heading for cover. As the raindrops intensified, Jessie shivered not so much from being cold as from the increasing sensation on her warm flesh. She watched the comical exodus of the sunbathers running for cover as the tropical rains were unleashed from the clouds overhead. Forty or so people gathered around the bar, crowding their swimsuit-clad bodies under the protection of a few feet of canopy.

Without thinking about it, Jessie followed as if she too would melt from the rain shower. She was drawn directly to where her husband stood at the bar, his eyes exploring her body. The surrounding people stood a respectful few inches from one another. Jessie and Rob could not hold back. Their bodies touched instantly, as if magnetically drawn together. The downpour continued, and the crowd talked and laughed. Jessie did not notice. Her senses were consumed by the warm tender touch of his fingers. The intensity was overwhelming. They spoke, but Jessie was unaware of what they were saying. As they touched, her desperation increased. Jessie felt a powerful urgency to consume him entirely, yet discretion held her back. She wanted her husband alone, entirely to herself, without the interested gazes of those around them. They ran through the rain without thinking, directly to their room. They entered, and immediately their lips met. The passionate journey in their long-term relationship began anew.

Jessie experienced an epiphany. She had discovered the passion within herself, recognizing her own needs and finding the inspiration to feed them. She learned that the instinct and desire for sex were already within her — she needed only to let them come out. Her search had ultimately brought her home again, and she found what was right in front of her the whole time. She simply needed to open her heart and mind to it. Jessie had finally summoned the passion *within* and was now on a never-ending quest with her lifelong mate.

CHAPTER SEVEN

THE JOURNEY HOME

REDIRECTING THE PASSION *WITHIN US*

WEATHERING THE QUEST FOR PASSION

Unlike Jessie's, Carla's passion flame has always burned brightly. She remembers strong impulses from a very early age. Carla was never uncomfortable with sex, and some might say she was too comfortable with it. In many ways she is at the opposite end of the spectrum from Jessie — that is, the Jessie that existed before her "awakening." Unlike Jessie, who had been sexually suppressed, Carla was, in a word, oversexed.

Though Jessie and Carla are very different from each other, they are alike in one important way: they both, for the first time, were recognizing that the problem was not so much what was missing in their relationship with their husbands but rather what had been missing inside themselves. The journey for each of them was a journey home — home to the passion within. Whether that meant discovering sexual desires for the first time or redirecting sexual focus, the result was a completion, an ending, a homecoming, and ultimately a beginning of a new and far more productive adventure — a lifelong passion quest with their mate.

Carla's Potentially Perilous Journey

In researching this book, I asked Carla to share her story with me. As we may recall, Carla waited longer than most to get married. She dated around and focused on her career — a real-life "Samantha" from *Sex and the City.* Although she had much sexual experience, she was by no means a slut. Her relationships were always monogamous — there were just a lot of them. She was what some refer to as a "serial monogamist."

When I made contact with her after a long absence, I was surprised to find that she had finally settled down and actually married someone. She had always sworn that she would never marry because she enjoyed dating too much. Nevertheless, Carla told me that when she married three years ago, she was more than ready to settle down. While all her friends were having babies, she had remained single and career oriented, but she had eventually come to depend on one particular boyfriend to always be there when she came home. Despite her attempts to drive him away, John had stayed put, so, finally, she agreed to marry him.

As we discussed in chapter 5, Carla and John's marriage began passionately enough, but eventually routine crept into the bedroom. Carla thought she was simply missing the excitement of first-time sex with new and different partners. John's willing-ness to discuss sex with a third party was exciting and possibly even fueling her desire to go out and conquer someone new. We may remember that Carla's travel schedule provided plenty of opportunity to carry out this wish. She considered tales from other women who claimed that their affair actually added a spark to their long-term relationship. Carla, however, could never lie to her husband. She had never cheated on any man and was not about to start now.

We know that in this particular case, John was actually giv-ing Carla his permission. The two were in fact discussing him *wanting* her to have a sexual encounter with another man. Even though John professed to be excited about hearing the details, Carla recognized that her husband could end up regretting his decision. Jealousy and anger could take hold, and she would feel guilty. The situation seemed complicated and not worth the risks. Ultimately, Carla thought, since she would be having "just sex," the "reward" would certainly not be worth hurting John or even destroying her marriage.

As I listened to Carla's story, I thought the issue sounded settled. Carla logically saw pitfalls involved in making this fan-tasy a reality, so she should avoid it. Why was she still discussing it? Why was she not letting it go?

I asked Carla some pointed questions, encouraging her to tell me more about her sexual past and what she thought this "fantasy" would fulfill. Carla expressed a strong physical yearn-ing for the heat of a new encounter. First-time sex was a drug, and she was drawn to it. Too long now she had sworn it off, but still it haunted her. When temptation presented itself, she struggled to resist. How could she not take her husband up on his offer? The fantasies were consuming her. She needed a fix.

A Journey into the Past

When Carla was only sixteen, her mother took her to a gynecologist so that Carla could be placed on birth control pills. Carla did not have a boyfriend, nor was she sexually active. Her mother explained, however, that the pills were a preemptive measure. Unfortunately her mother did not spend any time discussing sex with Carla, setting any boundaries, or parenting her on this topic in any meaningful way.

Carla, on the other hand, thought that taking birth control pills was "very cool" and felt very grown up. She had not even qualified for her driver's license yet, but she was now "licensed" for sex. For this license, however, she did not have to pass a test, and she had received no training, no warnings, no lectures — nothing. Carla was put behind the wheel without an education.

As a result, she learned about sex the hard way. Carla wasted no time after her visit to the doctor. She badly wanted a boyfriend and approval. Carla found that, with no worries about getting pregnant, she had the freedom to use whatever means necessary to get the acceptance she longed to receive. Unfortunately she crashed many times, but being so young, her injuries — at least on the outside — healed quickly.

I first met Carla in college. In the uptight environment of the private, Midwestern religious institution we attended, Carla stood out as the most openly sincere and genuine person I had ever known. She was always ready to party and always eager to be included, but she often felt left out. Carla was and is beautiful, but she did not realize it. She recognized her appeal to men but never really felt attractive. Many people treated her poorly because of the defenses she had set up to protect herself, partly because of the way she looked.

Carla was never really interested in the nice guys who were

gaga over her and would dote on her. Sometimes they represented a temporary ego-boosting fix, but they were no challenge. Carla loved the bad boys — the ones whom she had to chase and conquer. They were not always "bad" per se, just hard to get — the harder, the better.

For Carla, however, the challenge was rarely in getting them into bed — that was usually easy. Rather, the challenge was in making them like and want her, *really* want her. Love was an even bigger challenge. Carla was always "in love" and determined to make that "high" mutual, despite the fact that the men she chose were not remotely interested in loving her.

Carla did not have many female friends — at least, not close ones. She seemed to depend heavily on her boyfriend of the moment. She would invariably profess not to need a man, but her actions told a different story. When she was without a boyfriend, she would quickly and actively work on finding a new one.

During this time in college, I remember meeting Carla's mother. I often encountered her at the beginning or end of a semester or at a sorority event. She was critical of everyone and everything, but especially of Carla. I recall once when our dorm floor monitor complimented Carla in front of her mother, telling Carla how beautiful she was. Carla's mother quickly and tartly responded, "Do not tell her that. She might actually believe such a tale." Carla felt that her good grades, appearance, part-time jobs to help pay for school, charity work, and choice in boyfriends would never be good enough in her mother's eyes.

Carla's father, regrettably, was rarely around. According to Carla, even when he was there, he was emotionally unavailable. Nevertheless, Carla adored him and would try hard to get his attention.

Twenty years later, Carla described her relationship with her parents as the textbook example of the critical mother, the distant father, and the kid who just wanted their love and approval. Carla told me that she never sought help from a therapist or tried to psychoanalyze the effect her relationship with her parents had on shaping her needs and interactions with men. She did say, however, that continually trying to fill herself up and affirm her self-worth through her relationships with men had resulted in a series of emotionally based bad decisions about intimacy. She just wanted to feel desired and be needed.

Internal Explorations — Traveling Without the Necessary Luggage

With marriage, all the rules had changed for Carla. She knew her husband loved her. She knew he would always be there for her. This should have been all the reassurance she would ever need, but still she wasn't satisfied. She was drawn to the contest, the chase. She had a need to continually feel that self-confirming high, proving that she was desirable.

In marriage, the chase was over. Carla had already "conquered" her husband. The constant validation of her abilities, her beauty, and her talent was no longer as readily available as it had been in her continual string of new, passionate affairs. She had found "the one" and he loved her. Sometimes he was a challenge, but the conquering was over.

Winning her husband's affections completely was still not enough. Once he became so human to her, he no longer fed her need for validation. Carla was still seeking to fill herself up externally, but now that she and John were so emotionally connected and intimate, the "external" became not just outside herself but outside her marriage as well.

How would she now find that confirmation and reassurance? How was she to obtain the rush of the conquests that marked her dating journeys? How was she to refocus her need for self-confirming new encounters? The passion was already there within her, but the focus was misdirected. It was as if she had started off on a passion quest but lacked the necessary luggage to make the journey. What was missing inside Carla could potentially make for a perilous expedition.

DISCOVERING THE TRUE VALUE OF TRAVELING TOGETHER

Sometimes the solution is not to awaken the passion within or to rediscover it but rather to *redirect* it.

One night, when the fantasy came so close to happening, a light came on inside Carla. She was out of town on business. Carla had finished her work and was having a nightcap alone in the hotel bar. A stranger approached her. He was young, well dressed, and attractive. Carla was working on her second martini (not to mention the wine she had at dinner), and instead of dismissing him, she responded with some harmless banter. He was charming and shamelessly flirtatious. She was about to call it a night when he leaned in to kiss her. Carla hesitated but briefly kissed him back. It was indeed a passionate kiss, but it did not feel right. It was nothing like the fantasy — all hot and out of control. At that moment, Carla wanted only to touch her husband and feel *his* hot breath on her neck. So, with a quick excuse, she stood up and rushed away to the safety of her room.

Carla was on the phone with John before she even shut the door. Tears flooded her eyes. She realized right then and there that John was all the man she needed or wanted. She knew that it would never feel right with another man. The fantasy was exciting and arousing, but it was just a fantasy. Maybe the reality would be great for someone else, but it was not great for her — not even close.

What had happened to her in those telling moments when she had the opportunity to make fantasy a reality? What had become of her need for validation and reassurance and the rush of the conquest? Where had her urgent need for a sexual fix gone? Carla told me that, in addition to feeling just plain wrong, the near encounter seemed hollow. The man had been very charming and sexy, but the "passionate" kiss was not even close to the depth she felt with John. I suggested to Carla that perhaps extramarital sexual encounters would always seem hollow because they lacked the one thing she never possessed until now: the depth of love and intimacy that she shared with John — the feeling of complete acceptance.

These emotions were new to Carla. She had heard that women who waited longer to be married had a much lower divorce rate — and in her heart she knew why. Having spent a lot of time alone, having been single so long, Carla valued and fully recognized the benefits of the companionship that John offered her. But her sudden realization *was so much more than that* — so much more than just acknowledging companionship. Carla now understood that she was okay — that she really was loved and accepted and did not need continual validation.

This was a defining moment for Carla. She recognized the power within herself. Carla had the ability to *control* her passions and direct them in meaningful and productive ways.

This realization was not the end, though. It was instead a turning point. Carla still recognized the strong passionate tendencies within her, but now she felt empowered to redirect those passions in a way that felt comfortable and right for her relationship with John.

How would Carla accomplish this? How could she feed her strong passionate nature and reignite the heat that she felt in the beginning of the relationship — and then keep that feeling alive? There is no one right answer to these questions but rather a plethora of possibilities within the confines of a monogamous relationship — possibilities that Carla had not envisioned before.

She now recognized how her attitude was contributing to the idea that the passion in her relationship had been waning. She thought she missed being with someone new and different, but at this point she realized that "new and different" did not have to mean a new and different *person*. Such a perilous route seemed the easy way to an exciting sexual encounter, but Carla now knew that the simple path was not the awe-inspiring journey she longed to be on. In fact, it felt more like a dead end. She had experienced that path so many times before. The real excitement came not from a new mate but rather from the ever-growing and ever-changing journey with John. This was a much deeper and more meaningful exploration.

The depth of her intimate relationship with John put her on a whole new path — one she now recognized as more exciting and eventful than the series of shallow encounters she was accustomed to in her single life. The journey with John was certainly not for the faint of heart, nor was it for those averse to risk — but it did, in its own way, have a sense of security that no ordinary safety net could provide.

This journey would require more effort and commitment than had anything else in her life, but she would find that the sights she would see and the pleasures she and her husband would discover together would be worth the occasional blood, sweat, and tears.

Sublimation and Satisfaction

Carla's attitude was only one piece of the puzzle. The journey required sublimation as well. Emotionally, Carla could no longer envision a reality that included sexual encounters with other men. However, Carla's sense of adventure — and her physical yearnings — did not evaporate. The redirection of her passions involved not just reducing or otherwise fulfilling her need for validation but also sublimating her passionate nature and strong sexual yearnings. How would she accomplish this?

Carla found the answer by accident. While on vacation with her husband at an all-inclusive resort, she discovered the thrill of "dangerous" adventures. John and Carla met a couple who encouraged them to rise off the beach blanket and try out the resort's many sporting activities. Over the course of the week, John and Carla tried rock climbing, hang gliding, body surfing, scuba diving, and swimming with sharks.

Carla found a new "high." The thrill of trying out something different, and sharing that experience with John, was as exciting, inspiring, and addictive to her as any sexual escapade she had ever encountered. This was not a case of giving up one addiction for another but rather finding alternatives to sublimate her passions. These alternatives did not replace sex but instead provided a means to further share her energies and passionate nature with her mate, to feel more complete and fulfilled, and to not have to sacrifice her needs in order to be successful in her monogamous, long-term relationship.

Additionally, and equally as important, these daring but nonsexual activities gave her a high that easily translated into excitement in the bedroom. When John and Carla would return to their hotel room after reaching the top of the rock or feeling the exhilaration of gliding through the air, they would then join in an experience together that Carla described as "profoundly earth-shattering sex."

The adrenaline rush they would receive from the daring or challenging activity would produce a natural and even sexual high. For them, it was a fabulous form of foreplay. The awesome rush from the sport would culminate in their ripping off each other's clothes and finishing the "high" from the challenge they had just accomplished. Exhausted in the best possible way, Carla and John would then collapse in each other's arms — satisfied and peacefully complete.

Redirecting the Passion Within

> By feeding the sexual intimacy in our long-term relationship, we are not taking away from one priority to give to another but rather positively affecting all our priorities and exponentially increasing the passion we have for all things in life.

Carla found the means within herself to redirect her passions. She escaped her pattern of "serial monogamy" and found a way to reduce and refocus her need for validation. Carla was fortunate to finally recognize her overdependence on sex and to eventually learn how to sublimate her strong desires. Instead of experiencing a series of superficial relationships, she is on a new journey with her mate, rediscovering pleasures and reaching greater depths of intimacy in her long-term relationship. Her passion quest with her husband is not slowing down; it is just heating up.

Carla became the subject of many conversations among my girlfriends. This fascination was due in part to the inability of some women (especially those consumed by taking care of children and/or advancing their career) to even comprehend such a sexually passionate nature in a person. However, there are many women out there who are going much farther than Carla did: they are having affairs; dancing on tables; dating married men; participating in unconventional sex; frequenting "adult" parties, clubs, and resorts; etc. Carla's "nature" pales in comparison.

The lessons Carla learned about redirecting her passions may be helpful to women who are struggling to fulfill their strong sexual and passionate nature within the confines of their monogamous relationships. But whether we can identify with Carla or not, there is worthy "travel advice" in her story for all of us. Carla's experiences provide meaningful lessons even for those who neither identify with Carla's strong sexual appetite nor come close to comprehending her use of sex to validate her self-worth.

> Do we redirect and exhaust our passionate urges and desires to such an extent that we harm the very depth and intimacy of our most important long-term relationship?

We all need to take a look at the ways in which *we* may misdirect, misuse, or even use up our passionate and innate urges and needs. Maybe we possess sexual needs as strong as Carla's, and maybe we do not, but we are nevertheless constantly pouring energy and passion into many things and many people. We take on countless roles and responsibilities. We spread ourselves thin and then feel as if we never have enough time to get anything done. We are the ones filling up our schedules and devoting our time and energies to all these tasks. Would it benefit our health and the health of our relationship to place some of that energy and commitment into a quest for passion with our mate?

The time and energy we put into a quest for passion with our long-term mate will produce *more* energy, *not* burn it up.

One woman commented that, unlike Carla, she does not have excess passion to redirect. Instead she feels as if she does not have enough to go around. Putting more energy into seeking passion with her mate would mean taking time away from her children and her career. Many of us are able to identify with this woman's thoughts. But remember, by feeding the sexual intimacy in our long-term relationship, we are not taking away from one priority to give to another but rather positively affecting all our priorities and exponentially increasing the passion we have for all things in life.

To redirect passion, we must recognize that the passion exists within us and needs only to be channeled into our lifelong journey with our mate. As adults we often forget that we *need* to enjoy ourselves. This is not selfish but is a necessary part of maintaining good mental and physical health so that we may not simply function in all our roles and responsibilities but actually perform them at superior levels.

The time and energy we put into a quest for passion with our long-term mate will produce *more* energy, *not* burn it up. Pleasure, fun, and relaxation are energizing. We will have more of what we need to be a better partner in our relationship, as well as a better parent, professional, and person because we will be calmer, happier, and more fulfilled.

If our innate sexual needs and those of our mate are being met, then the children, the family as a whole, and even our career will reap the healthy benefits. Committing ourselves to seek passion brings pleasure and closeness that only such sexual intimacies with our mate can produce. This makes for a more stable and emotionally committed marriage, and our children will benefit from witnessing such a relationship. We know that they are learning how to love and be loved by watching us.

Our careers will also benefit because, when we are at work, we will be better able to focus on our *work*. Something exciting and fun, something pleasurable and relaxing to look forward to when we get home, makes the day's work a little easier. Many times in literature and in life, people have said that they are more productive and more creative when they are in a stable relationship, having great or even just good sex. We are not distracted. We are not tempted. We are where we should be.

The passion must come from within.

The passion journey we choose to take with our mate will be different from anyone else's. There is no right way to seek and maintain the passion — there is only the way that makes sense for us and our relationship. But what makes sense to us will only result in a successful journey if we first take a look inside ourselves — not at what is missing in our relationship with our spouse but at what might be missing inside us. Whether that means discovering the passion for the first time, as Jessie did, or redirecting and channeling its focus into an ultimately far more productive and energizing adventure with our mate, the passion must come from within. If it does, the journey together has the best chance of providing a lifetime of passionate discoveries.

CHAPTER EIGHT

WILD EXPLORATIONS

WHEN OUTSIDERS JOIN THE JOURNEY . . .
AND OTHER RISKY SPORTS

When I started talking to friends, acquaintances, and visitors to my Web site about their sexual experiences, I was surprised by the incredible spectrum of possibilities for exploration. Many had decided to try something different, something creative and even taboo, and when they reported their results to me, I began to realize that the extent of wild explorations I was to uncover would be more far-reaching than I had imagined. Once my conversations with people became more intimate, I learned that in fact much has been undertaken in the name of passion, some paths productive and some not so productive. Even where I live, in the relatively conservative Midwest, sexual experimentation among married couples is prevalent, and my research has shown that many of those who are not experimenting wish they were.

So many times we hear about a couple divorcing and comment about how there was no outward evidence of unhappiness. We often hear, "They seemed like such a happy couple." I have commented in doing my research, "My, what a conservative couple they appear to be, and yet look at their wild approach to their sex life." Or "My, how 'into' each other they always seem and how unhappy and bored they are with their sex life." In paying attention to people, I have found that the things I thought I knew were often wrong, and the things I uncovered about people I thought I knew were astonishing. The most interesting and sordid personal accounts that I have collected have come from people who, on the surface, are upright, law-abiding, neighborly, churchgoing folks.

I discovered that more couples than I had ever imagined were open to adventurous journeys or had already experimented with them. Often in long-term relationships one or both partners think about, fantasize about, or even propose experimentation of an unconventional nature, such as three-ways or swinging or even kinky sex play. Some, of course, never act on the impulse and simply fantasize instead. Somewhat surprising, though, is how often the female partner suggests, and wants to possibly seek out, experimentation of this nature.

One acquaintance of mine, whom I will call Rachael, in fact admitted in confidence that she and her husband have been part of the "swinging" crowd for nearly three years. I was surprised. I had an image in my mind of what swingers were like, and Rachael and her husband did not fit my impression. They seemed like such a conservative, traditional couple. I would never have found out had I not been researching this book. People apparently put a lot of effort into keeping the "lifestyle" confidential, and couples who really swing do not talk about it. My friend Dan always suggests at parties that the guys throw their keys into a bowl, with the idea of selecting a different set when they leave (the implication being that each would leave with someone else's wife). Dan, however, is all talk. I began to realize that my image of the kind of people who swing was not only inaccurate but naive as well. There is no stereotypical swinger. I have found that the couples we suspect of swinging may not, and the ones we do not suspect of swinging might actually be involved.

I have gathered information from my Web site, other sites, and books on the topic of wild exploration. The details I have acquired from these sources have been helpful and have filled in a lot of blanks, but the best sources of information have been the many people I have met in my travels, and all the Passion Seekers and acquaintances who have shared their stories and answered my questions. As we popped the corks on many a bottle of wine, friends both old and new revealed real-life experiences in detail, often while the adrenaline was still flowing and, in some instances, so were the tears.

In listening to Passion Seekers and other acquaintances, I have uncovered the details of some passion journeys that have, accidentally in many cases, turned into some wild explorations. These are actual journeys taken by people just like us. Their stories may reflect experiences we or people we know have had, or may reflect something we have only thought of or fantasized about. For some, the experiences may be food for thought as they find themselves venturing down similar paths. The curious and inexperienced might find these explorations fascinating. Still others may be shocked and feel that conventional, upstanding citizens do not condone such actions. Whatever our opinion on the subject, the reality remains that more and more couples are experimenting and struggling to spice things up in the bedroom.

Maybe we will see something we thought we wanted to try, but after reading about it, we will think twice. Or maybe we will see something we now wish to explore, and from witnessing the trials and tribulations of those who have already journeyed there, we will be better prepared. In reading about these experiences, we may prevent some real heartache and find our way with less embarrassment and less marital discord. It is not necessary to blindly stumble down the path or seek a journey without preparation when the experienced can tell us what we need to know. These real-life examples can help us find our *own* way toward a more fulfilling and passionate sex life in our long-term relationship, whether we choose "wild explorations" or more tame ones.

COURTNEY'S QUEST

Courtney had experimented with a woman once when she was in college. Courtney was, at the time, "bi-curious" (interested in knowing what it would be like to have a same-sex encounter). She recalls (although at the time she was under the influence of quite a lot of a fraternity's "purple passion punch") that it was all very hot and exciting. She liked the soft feel of the girl's skin and the tenderness of her touch. Her boyfriend, who witnessed the experience, apparently really enjoyed it as well, but afterward he started questioning Courtney's sexual preferences. They soon broke up. It was very awkward, and she lost not only her boyfriend over the encounter but also the friendship of her girl-friend.

Many years have passed since Courtney's college experience. She married about four years after graduation, and a few years after that, she had the first of her three children. She is currently a stay-at-home mom with an extremely busy schedule, taking care of everyone. Courtney told me that although she was not really bored with her sex life, she longed for the early heated days with her husband. Before children and with a lot more time on their hands, Courtney and her mate were extremely playful sexually. They tried different positions and locations. They shared a few sex toys, books, and videos. They enjoyed each other often and effortlessly. Now Courtney felt as if she really, really had to work at it.

Courtney and her husband tried many of the techniques set out in different sex-help books. They found a few fun tips, but for the most part they thought the information was obvious, redundant, and in some cases just plain ridiculous. Courtney was beginning to think that there was nothing left to explore. Although she incorrectly thought she had little choice but to just get used to the mediocrity of sex with the same person for the rest of her married life, she was still searching for a way to spice things up. She began fantasizing about unconventional sexual methods.

After about four years of marriage, Courtney's husband was the first one to bring the idea of a threesome out into the open. He suggested that it might be fun if they brought another person into their bed and shared the experience. At first, Courtney felt her husband was clearly not satisfied by having sex with just her. Despite the fact that she was actually entertaining similar thoughts, she was angry and hurt that her mate would suggest such a thing. Then she worried that if she did not go along with his suggestion he might go out and have an affair. She thought he was perhaps already contemplating such a thing, and his "suggestion" was a last-ditch effort to include her in his desire to have sex with someone else.

Courtney decided to go along with the idea and at least show interest in it. It was always possible that a willing participant might never come along anyway. For a while, talking about the possibility of a three-way was great foreplay, and Courtney was even finding that the fantasy was starting to turn her on. The only thing that kept haunting her was the experience she had in college. What if they brought another woman into their bedroom and Courtney had a great time with the woman? Would her husband question her sexuality? What if the reality of the experience was not as good as the fantasy? Would it be worth the risks?

There were a million other questions in Courtney's mind. Could she bear the idea of her husband intimately touching another woman, let alone actually seeing him have intercourse with her? What if he ended up enjoying this other woman more than he enjoyed her, his own wife? What if he wanted to see this woman again? And what about their safety? One advantage to being in a completely monogamous relationship was that they never had to worry about sexually transmitted diseases.

Courtney decided that, if they were really going to do this, there had to be some ground rules. First, she told her husband, the encounter would have to happen on vacation, somewhere out of town. This, in her mind, solved the problem of having to see this other person again. Also, she felt that the anonymity of a different city would ensure that no one they knew would ever find out what they had done.

Second, Courtney decided that the only way her ego could handle the experience was if the other woman was not as good-looking as she was. Courtney thought that if she felt more attractive, she would not feel as threatened by the other woman and therefore not feel at risk of losing her mate. She knew logically that she would not likely lose her husband, but her youthful insecurities still, at times, got the better of her.

Despite the preparation, when it actually happened, Courtney was not the least prepared. While on vacation, Courtney and her husband were at a bar at their resort when a woman started talking to her husband. The young woman smiled warmly at Courtney, and she did not feel threatened at all. It was actually Courtney who asked the woman to go to the resort's Jacuzzi with them. Once there, in the dark of the Jacuzzi, things started getting hot. Courtney touched the woman under the water, and the next thing she knew the woman and Courtney's husband were passionately kissing. Courtney was so turned on by the sight that she did not feel even a pang of jealousy.

Back in their hotel room and much to Courtney and her husband's surprise, the woman was all over Courtney. Courtney's husband could have left the room and would not have been noticed. Courtney did not completely forget about him, though. In fact, she brought him into the action and even encouraged the woman to go all the way with him. In the heat of the moment all of Courtney's inhibitions about her husband touching the other woman, let alone going all the way, were gone. In fact, the sight of her husband pleasing this other woman was extremely erotic to Courtney.

She woke up the next morning with not only a physical hangover but an emotional one as well. All the feelings of jealousy that she thought she had conquered the night before came rushing over her. And she was angry — angry that she had pushed her husband to go all the way with the woman, angry that he did not refuse despite her urging him, and angry that she enjoyed it so much. It was all very confusing. All she could think about was how relieved she was that the woman was checking out of the resort that day and that no one else knew how extremely naughty she had been. Courtney would never have to see the woman again, but she did have to face her husband. Unfortunately, she found in him an easy target with which to let loose with the bulk of her confused emotions.

Courtney wanted to blame her husband. It was his idea, after all, and he went along with everything that happened. He even took her up on her offer when she urged him to have intercourse with the woman. The reality she had yet to realize was that she had taken a leadership role in the experience. She had encouraged both her husband and the woman to have sex, and Courtney got exactly what she wanted, or thought she wanted, at the time. It had been so exciting, so thrilling, and it had felt so good.

After a few tears and a little time, and, most important, the continued devotion of her husband, Courtney was able to process what had happened and not attribute more meaning to it than was warranted. In fact, the experience eventually became a continued source of erotic stimulation whenever she and her husband discussed or otherwise recalled that passionate evening on their last vacation.

A few years later, the opportunity arose again. This time the woman befriended Courtney first but then actually suggested the three-way to her husband while Courtney was in the ladies' room. Courtney was much more aware of the other woman than she was in the previous encounter. She wanted to make sure that this woman would enjoy herself, at least as much as Courtney and her husband would. Courtney realized that, having "faked it" a few times herself, there was no real way to know if their guest was being properly taken care of.

She encouraged her husband to try using his "mouth technique" on the woman. Courtney tried doing to the woman all the things that she herself liked, but she knew that her own preferences in the bedroom were ever changing. How was she to ensure that this woman was really enjoying herself, and how would she know if this other person had an orgasm? Courtney tried to go on the noises the woman was making and increase or change the manipulation accordingly. Her neck was cramping up, not to mention her fingers. It seemed to be an arduous task. Where exactly was this woman's G-spot? Courtney had a new-found appreciation for what it must be like for a man to try to please a woman.

After the encounter, Courtney discussed her concerns with her husband. He could not understand why she cared so much. He pointed out that they had done what they could for their guest and questioned why Courtney was worried about it anyway since they were never going to see this woman again. He agreed that a lot of effort goes into trying to make a woman experience orgasm, but for him there was a clear limit to his concern about a person he had no relationship with. This comment made Courtney realize the complete lack of emotion involved in the event for her husband. His only concern was for Courtney and her peace of mind. Realizing this, Courtney felt even closer to him and was able to look at this encounter as something they had shared together for their mutual pleasure — and nothing more.

As time passed, Courtney again began to feel the need to crank things up a notch in the bedroom, but where to go from here? Could their relationship weather yet another unconventional attempt to spice things up? Would the third time be a charm? Or were the floodgates now open? Maybe another three-way with a woman would not be enough — for either of them. Did they need to again try to find something different?

Courtney began thinking about what it would be like to have a man join them this time. When she finally suggested this to her husband, Courtney was shocked by his reaction. His homophobic fears aside, the green-eyed monster had taken hold of him. There appeared to be a double standard. Courtney could not understand why this suggestion was any different than the one her husband had made when he wished to have another woman in their bed. Nevertheless, he was emphatic that there was a difference, but he could not seem to clearly delineate why.

One thing he did express, in no uncertain terms, was how uncomfortable he would be with another naked man in the room with them, let alone in their bed. The possibility of Courtney's husband actually coming into physical contact with the other man was too much for him. Even with Courtney in the middle of them, the risk was too great that their flesh might accidentally touch. These comments were surprising to Courtney, who had never heard her husband utter anything homophobic in all their time together. Apparently this proposed scene would cross the line for him.

Courtney's husband was perplexed by her request. He seemed to think he was all the man she should ever want. Maybe, Courtney thought, her husband was just as worried, if not more so, about losing her as she had been about losing him. At first, she felt that her husband's objections were unfair and that he was just going to have to deal with the situation the way she had to. What is good for the goose is good for the gander. It was, after all, *her* turn, and she deserved it.

At this point Courtney confided in her close girlfriends. She was really starting to resent the fact that her husband could not do for her what she had done for him on *two* separate occasions. Courtney felt entitled. After trying out his idea, she thought it was time to have something her way. How were they going to get past this?

Courtney's experiences thus far can be helpful to others for a number of reasons. Discussions with Courtney and those in the know reveal universal issues that must be considered before inviting a "guest" into bed. These issues are exposed by asking the following questions:

Traveling with a Third Party — Questions to Ask Yourself *Before* Such a Wild Exploration

- Have you considered the extent of physical contact with the outsider that you are comfortable with, and are you going to be okay if, during the heat of the moment, that line is crossed by you or your partner?
- Are you prepared to see your mate excited about/for someone else? Are you prepared to share this excitement and be happy for his pleasure?
- Do you believe your mate is comfortable with seeing you excited about/for someone else and will happily share in this with you?
- Is the thought of this experience creating any feelings of insecurity? Do either of you frequently or even occasionally battle feelings of jealousy? If so, then consider whether your relationship is secure enough to share a sexually intimate encounter with an outsider.
- Finally, is this something that really interests you, or are you just going along with it because it is what your mate wants?

As for Courtney and her quest to keep the passion flame alive in her relationship, we will have to read on. Will they invite another outsider into their bedroom? Will Courtney get a male guest? Or will they try something else to crank things up a notch next time? Through discussions with girlfriends about their passion quests, Courtney may just find a way through her own wild expedition. We will revisit her in chapter 9. Now, however, is a good time to share Lisa's story.

LISA'S QUEST

Lisa is very outgoing but is considered by most to have a fairly conservative mind-set. She regularly attends church and considers herself a religious person. Lisa was a professional career woman for a number of years, but after her second child was born, she gave up the job to "be there" for her children. Now she is an extremely active stay-at-home mom and is always volunteering for something, including many fund-raisers for worthy causes. One "cause," though, that she had lost touch with was her passion for sex with her husband.

Lisa had never done anything sexually that one would consider "wild." She and her husband had what Lisa described as "mediocre" sex at best. The only time the sex was really good was when they were on vacation. On a trip alone with her husband, Lisa said, all her other roles, especially that of motherhood, were not consuming her energy and her desire. She was able to be completely "there" in the moment with her husband. Lisa longed to find a way to have "vacation sex" more often than once a year.

Lisa's quest seeking the missing passion took her on a wild expedition into a great and vast unknown land — the land of swingers. It happened quite by accident.

Lisa and her husband were staying in Las Vegas at a fancy hotel for the weekend. Lisa was alone poolside while her husband courted clients at a nearby convention. A group of very happy partyers had just camped out in the cabana next to Lisa's. While she sipped a margarita, Lisa could hear them talking and laughing, but from her vantage point she could not see them. The conversation was loaded with intelligent banter, sexual innuendo, and extremely flirtatious remarks. They were obviously a close group of friends who were quite comfortable with one another.

Hoping to satisfy her curiosity by getting a look at this group, Lisa came out of her cabana and headed toward the pool for a quick dip. On her way back, she caught the eye of an attractive man in the group who was giving a massage to one of the ladies. The woman he was massaging looked up and smiled and asked Lisa if she would like to join them for a drink. Lisa accepted and suddenly found herself welcomed into the midst of this warm and generous group of people.

There were three couples sprawled out among the lounge chairs around the cabana. One couple was sharing a chair with the woman lying back on her companion. Another couple was in the shade of the cabana, snacking at a tableful of fruits and cheeses. The gentleman who had first caught Lisa's eye, a man named Rick, made the introductions. It was then that Lisa realized she was not in Kansas anymore.

The women were not paired off with their respective spouses, and the touching taking place was not like any she had ever encountered with the husbands of her friends. Could they be swingers? Lisa's impression was quickly confirmed when Rick asked her if she and her husband had ever swung before. Lisa's curiosity again got the better of her, and although she readily admitted her ignorance of the "lifestyle," she professed to be very interested.

Lisa learned a lot from her afternoon in the sun with her newfound friends. The recipient of Rick's massage was a woman named Sarah. Sarah was a petite blonde with a kind and inviting smile. She took it upon herself to educate Lisa with the story of how she became a swinger.

Sarah's tale began with an admission that she and her

husband, Tom, had been doing everything they thought possible to keep the fires burning in their relationship. They were both of an adventurous nature, with a passion for good wine and stimulating conversation. One evening while waiting for a table at the bar of a newly opened hot spot, they met a couple. The female was very attractive in a dark, exotic sort of way, and she had a laugh that drew Sarah in. The woman invited Sarah and her husband to a private party at a nearby hotel. After dinner and without hesitation, Sarah and Tom went to the hotel to check out this party.

The party turned out to be for couples only, and the atmosphere was steamy. Loud music played as a sexily clad crowd gave new meaning to the words "dirty dancing." The exotic woman's husband came over and started talking to Sarah while Tom was getting drinks at the bar. He professed to be an endocrinologist, and he and his wife were in town just to attend this event. He told Sarah how beautiful and sexy she looked as he played with her with his eyes. The beat of the music, the wine she had drunk at dinner, and the attentions of this attractive and interesting man put Sarah in a state. She did not object when he pulled her out onto the dance floor and held her close. She felt his hot breath in her ear as he caressed her with soft words. An extremely intense and heated kiss ensued. Sarah now had but one thought, and that was to be alone with this man.

As Sarah exited the dance floor, she caught Tom watching from the bar. He was standing next to the doctor's wife. She was smiling up at him, but the look on Tom's face was not a happy one. Sarah's dance companion whispered into her ear, asking that she and Tom accompany him and his wife to their room. Sarah wanted desperately to do so, with or without her husband. She was feeling very naughty and, despite the disapproving look on her husband's face, was going to find a way to continue the fun with this sexy couple.

Sarah pulled her husband aside and suggested that they continue the party alone with this pair in their hotel room upstairs. Tom was hesitant and uncertain. Sarah was persistent. Finally, Tom told her to go on ahead and he would be up there in a few minutes. Without further hesitation and with great sexual anticipation, Sarah rushed off with the couple.

After much heated interaction between Sarah and her new-found friends, Tom finally showed up. He was fairly intoxicated and seemed willing to interact. So Sarah motioned for the woman to approach. As Tom appeared to be involved with the woman, Sarah found her opportunity to interact alone with her doctor. As the action got heated on both sides of the large bed, Tom kept looking over at Sarah. She was really enjoying herself, and this became a problem for him. Before too long, the fun was over, and Tom quickly said good-bye and drew his wife out of the room.

The car ride home was quiet, too quiet. Sarah's nerve endings were still on fire, and her mind was cloudy. She did not know what to say. She knew that Tom was not all right with what had happened. When they got home, Tom grabbed Sarah and pushed her down on the bed. The sex was urgent and heated but with a dark and angry edge to it. Once Tom was satisfied, he rolled over and went to sleep without a word. Sarah was still on edge. The intensity of her sexual urges that night haunted her mind, and her heart still beat a rapid pulse.

The storm came long before morning. Tom was angry. The sight of his Sarah enraptured and impassioned by another man infuriated him and sexually aroused him at the same time. He could not organize his thoughts. He could not seem to understand the dichotomy of his emotions. He was overwhelmed.

Sarah, on the other hand, was frustrated. Tom was the one who always pressed for new adventure. He was the one who would often share fantasies about sex with others. Tom was not an insecure person, yet he seemed overwhelmed with jealousy.

Sarah also felt guilt — guilt that she so quickly and without hesitation became single-minded in her pursuit of this interaction, guilt that she enjoyed it so much, and guilt that she so readily discounted her husband's hesitations and pursued her goal regardless. She so easily had gotten swept up in the moment and had put aside the feelings of the one person she cared about most.

Sarah and Tom were not "all right" for some time after this encounter. However, in the dark of the night, their interactions became passionately intense whenever the event was recounted. Over time, their wounds healed and the pain was forgotten. All that was left was the sexual intensity that the memories elicited. Sarah could not articulate how it had worked out for them. It just had, and they somehow found their way back from the journey — together. Sarah felt fortunate.

Before too long, Tom began a subtle campaign to seek out further adventures on the swinging path. Despite how confident Tom was that he wanted to try it again, Sarah's scar still pained her, and she was not eager to repeat her mistake and cause the man she loved any more heartache. Nevertheless, with memories of the experience still lighting their fires at home, they eventually sought out another "party" to attend, and before they realized it, they started to share the "lifestyle." Their journey had begun again and was now never ending.

Sarah concluded her tale by telling Lisa that her first encounter happened seven years ago. Since that time, she and her husband had found their way with swinging, and it brought much *shared* pleasure into their committed life together. Sarah and Tom were now completely at peace with what she affectionately referred to as their "favorite hobby."

Sarah suggested to Lisa that she should consider the basic rules for swinging before she ever found herself stumbling, as Sarah had, in the heat of the moment. Sarah's rules were similar to the following:

Rules of the Road When "Traveling" in Groups

- First, be confident that you have a close relationship with your mate — one that is trusting, open, and honest.
- You must both be socially confident people who really enjoy sex and welcome new adventures.
- Make sure that you and your partner are on the same page. Discuss what actions and situations each of you are comfortable with and then stick to the plan.
- Both of you must agree on and be comfortable with the other couple selected. If one partner wants to back out or is otherwise hesitant, the situation is not right.
- When meeting other couples, never be pushy. Always take *no* for an answer. Coercion or pressuring is never acceptable.
- Remember that you and your partner are sharing the experience and are responsible for taking care of each other at all times, emotionally and otherwise.
- Try it — you might like it. Stop if it hurts.
- Never forget about your mate. Talk to each other, touch and otherwise maintain intimate contact, at least periodically, throughout the entire experience. Share it.
- Always consider your safety and reduce the risks.

When Lisa told a few of her close friends what she had heard about the swinging lifestyle, they listened with fascination. However, they professed to be somewhat shocked and appalled at the same time. For them, the idea was just too unconventional and immoral not to be outwardly condemned. But Lisa wondered if they secretly envied it. She knew she was beginning to. It seemed such an honest way to acknowledge those natural desires and sexual urges that were so secretly and dishonestly dealt with by people who cheated on their spouses, in mind or in body.

The swingers Lisa had met seemed so comfortable with their sexuality, and despite having sexual fun with outsiders, they each appeared to have a very close and intimate relationship with their mate. Sarah was emphatic that swinging was all about *sharing* with one's mate. Both parties agreed to it — no one lied or went behind anyone's back. Sarah and Tom said that over time they learned how to "be there" for each other during the encounters with other couples. They were on a shared journey that for them was always exciting and a source of never-ending fun.

Swingers make their lifestyle sound very natural and freeing and fun. Lisa realized, though, that the swinging experience was probably not always such a pleasant one. Sarah, in fact, admitted that she knew of couples who split over jealousies and insecurities that plagued their relationship following a sexual encounter with another couple. She explained that one's relationship with one's mate has to be very secure and comfortable. Complete openness and communication is vital, as it is in any sexual relationship. Regardless, complications can occur.

Sarah knew one couple who split up after the woman "fell in love" with someone else, someone with whom she and her husband had swung. Lisa questioned how easy it would be to emotionally detach from the sexual encounter even if one's spouse was present, "sharing" and "participating" nearby. Was she capable of always treating the encounters as "just sex" and nothing more? Would it be worth a try — worth the risk? Was it immoral to even think about or consider it?

We will soon find out whether Lisa's curiosity overcame her caution. For now, though, let us take a look at a few other wild explorations.

VARIOUS RISKY SPORTS

One wild exploration would be to venture into the world of BDSM (bondage, discipline, sadism, masochism). Before conducting research for this book, my understanding of this topic was limited because I could not comprehend how people could derive pleasure from pain.

So I began my research by reading the now classic *Story of O* by Pauline Réage, which caused quite a stir when it was widely discussed in the 1960s. The book is about a female fashion photographer from Paris who is kept locked up and blindfolded and is basically objectified. The fantasy is that of ultimate female submissiveness. Then I read the nineteenth-century classic *Venus in Furs* by Leopold von Sacher-Masoch, where the male character encourages his mistress to mistreat him. The word "masochism" is, in fact, derived from this author's name. These two novels do little to help one comprehend the more common uses of BDSM.

What did finally make an impact on me was the discovery that a girlfriend of mine professed to enjoy BDSM. I was at her house for a party and was sent upstairs to the master bedroom to use the bathroom. That bathroom was also occupied, so I found myself glancing at the book titles on the bookshelf as I waited. Being rather tall, I noticed some books on the top shelf, including several titles on the art of bondage and sadomasochism. My naïveté got the better of me, because I remember thinking that I had never seen Martha in black leather and certainly could not imagine her nerdy accountant husband tying her up or in any way "disciplining" her — or vice versa, for that matter.

After playing golf the next week, Martha and I had a long, private discussion over cocktails in the clubhouse. As usual, I received the best education from a friend with experience. Martha explained that BDSM came out of the closet (somewhat) in the 1960s and 1970s as a playful and fun sexual fantasy that, when conducted by completely willing participants, was an acceptable form of sexual pleasure. As a doctor, Martha explained that medically sadomasochism is not considered a disorder. Problems arise only when one's behavior is associated with a personality disorder or is otherwise negatively impacting important areas of social and occupational functioning within the realm of societal norms. There are still, she said, a lot of misconceptions about the common practices of BDSM, and therefore few admit to their involvement in it.

Martha explained that there is a BDSM subculture that advocates its safe practice among consensual adults as an actual "lifestyle." However, a large majority of participating couples are in committed relationships and use elements of BDSM only as occasional techniques to enhance their sexual encounters. Martha pointed out that "rough" sex itself, including "spanking" and "love biting," is sadomasochistic in nature. The practice of bondage, such as tying up our mate's wrists with a handkerchief, is commonplace. And, of course, many forms of sexual role-playing involve power exchanges common to BDSM play. The dominant/submissive theme is played out in such roles as doctor/patient and master/slave (see "Passion Seekers' Role-Playing Ideas" in chapter 4). Martha explained that many more couples than I had imagined had explored these and other forms of casual BDSM at some point in their relationship. Consensual BDSM play, she said, is making its way into the mainstream, providing an endless supply of variation and variety. As evidence of this, Martha pointed out that there are many adult stores and online suppliers of BDSM paraphernalia, as well as a number of books and videos on the subject.

Martha and her husband journeyed into BDSM after a trip to Japan. She told me that the practice is a lot more common in their culture, and her curiosity was stimulated by the visit. Martha recommended I read something more current on the subject, and she suggested a detailed book by Jay Wiseman entitled *SM 101: A Realistic Introduction.* This gave me a better understanding of the subculture and the acceptable forms of BDSM play.

Successful BDSM experimentation requires becoming educated in the rules of play and mastering some basics, including safety issues. Martha indicated that such preparation beforehand can result in some really intense sensations "like you never imagined." "Bondage" is the practice of tying someone up or otherwise restraining the person for *mutual* pleasure. Martha said that she and her husband take turns tying each other up. When she is in this position, her husband sexually teases her to the point of insanity, and her helplessness and his control over her are so erotic that she is able to achieve multiple orgasms of a "monumental nature." Imagine receiving *that* from a nerdy accountant (and I thought he only did taxes).

The common sadomasochistic activity of domination/submission involves a consensual power exchange in which one party derives sexual pleasure from controlling and even inflicting pain (and pleasure) and the other from submitting to it all. Martha has learned that the key for her and her mate is to establish rules in advance and to discuss everything before beginning. Complete trust in her "teammate" is required, and she knows that he always pays close attention to her limits. They have a "safeword" that the submissive partner can use to stop the play if the game goes too far and needs to end.

Martha pointed out that their occasional use of BDSM would not happen if they did not have a very secure and trusting relationship. She cautioned that there are wide spectrums of BDSM possibilities and that not all of them are safe or sane. Before venturing down this path, a clear understanding of the practice is important. Thanks to Martha, I have a better grasp of consensual mainstream forms of BDSM and can appreciate her and her husband's journey of wild exploration. I am happy that they have found a path that is fun, under the right circumstances, for them to venture down.

There are, of course, many other forms of wild explorations. "Exhibitionists," who derive sexual pleasure from being watched, and "voyeurs," who like to watch, are but two examples. When wild explorations are undertaken by *consenting* adults, our culture is becoming increasingly accepting. An acquaintance of mine admitted to me that she and her husband have some of their hottest sex in locations where they might get caught, and they have even had sex on the beach at a resort while in full view of those passing by — wow! Shocking what old married folks will do to spice things up.

> Concern for our partner must be our number one priority, or the purpose of improving the passion in our long-term relationship is defeated before play ever begins.

The journeys we have covered in this chapter are, for some couples, the answer to maintaining passion in a long-term relationship. These couples treat three-ways, swinging, BDSM, and other such activities not so much as wild explorations but rather as sports or hobbies. In these cases, sex becomes a team sport with rules of play. These rules need to be agreed upon in advance so that in the heat of the moment injuries do not occur. I am, of course, referring to emotional injuries, which could actually put your relationship out of play — permanently.

These extreme sports are not for the faint of heart. They are risky. Amateurs just learning the activity are at the greatest risk of stumbling and receiving serious injuries. Trust and complete confidence in our teammate is required. Nevertheless, even with preparation and a solid partner with whom we are comfortable and feel we can count on, the unexpected may occur, and the strength of our relationship with our teammate may be tested.

Sometimes actual participation in the sport may turn out to be a disappointment. In some cases, the sport may be better left as a fantasy. For example, using "imaginary playmates" (as discussed in chapter 4) may be a safer way for us to play the game, especially if we are the type to be easily (emotionally) injured.

If we wish to keep playing with our mate for years to come, we should always remember that hesitation for either partner means the game is over. We must heed the advice of Passion Seekers everywhere: concern for our partner must be our number one priority, or the purpose of improving the passion in our long-term relationship is defeated before play ever begins.

❦

CHAPTER NINE

THE JOURNEY WITH OUR MATE

SEEKING THE "PASSION POT OF GOLD" *WITHIN HIM*

Whether you have a "sporting nature" or whether you simply enjoy reading about the wild explorations of others, there are important messages within these titillating tales that will inspire us to take a closer look at our lifelong mate and rediscover the passion *within him.*

THE PASSION WITHIN OUR MATE

How much more can we learn about our mate if we really pay attention?

We return now to the real-life stories of Lisa and Courtney. These events are interesting from a voyeuristic perspective, but they also provide insight into exploring what we think is very familiar territory — our mate. The quote featured at the beginning of this book is particularly apropos here: "If you can awaken / inside the familiar / and discover it new / you need never / leave home." We shall see how this applies to any long-term relationship as we continue to follow Lisa and Courtney on their passion-seeking journeys. It is amazing what we may discover when we explore the ways in which we view our mate and the passion within *him*. Are we really paying attention? Do we need to take a new look at our spouse? Maybe we are working off of old or incorrect assumptions, thereby putting our quest for passion on the wrong track or throwing it off the track altogether.

> The human psyche is complex, and people are ever learning, growing, and changing. To stop paying attention is to wake up at some point next to a mate who is a virtual stranger.

When we last talked of Lisa, she was longing to find a way to have "vacation sex" more than once a year. She felt she was losing touch with her passion for making love to her mate and her passion for sex in general. The sex-help section of her local bookstore had been of little assistance, and she was beginning to show interest in exploring what in her world was considered unthinkable and taboo.

After her accidental meeting with a group of swingers in Las Vegas, Lisa had been thinking about the "lifestyle" a lot. She shared with her husband, Paul, the story she had been told that day at the hotel pool. Paul, like Lisa, was curious about the swinging lifestyle but also skeptical. The world in which they lived was very conservative, and such experimentation would be viewed in an extremely negative way. For them, the idea of living out such a fantasy did not seem realistic.

Lisa and Paul eventually found an answer, though. They took a journey seeking the passion and, in the process, rediscovered each other. In the end, Lisa said, she was given a unique opportunity to see her mate anew and, in doing so, reignited the passion in their relationship. She believes that her passion quest experiences truly transformed her and her relationship for the better, and she therefore insisted that I share her discoveries (with identifying information altered) in the hopes of helping all of us rediscover the passion that is within our mate.

When I began my discreet efforts to uncover what was going on *under* the covers in America's bedrooms, I learned a lot from women such as Lisa who were willing to share their personal journeys with me. However, never did I imagine the extent of what I would learn, not just about the endless spectrum of bedroom possibilities but also about myself — the way I looked at sex and sexuality, and especially the way I viewed sex with my long-term mate. Even after so many years with him, I am still learning more every day. One never really knows what someone else is thinking. The human psyche is complex, and people are ever learning, growing, and changing. To stop paying attention is to wake up at some point next to a mate who is a virtual stranger.

The events I uncovered both give us an opportunity to peek inside the neighbor's bedroom and inspire us to ignite the fires at home. But the stories will offer *so much more than that.* The eye-opening experiences of Lisa, Courtney, and others in this chapter show us just how much we can learn about our mate if we really pay attention. These women ultimately take a new and revealing look at their old partner. What they discover opens their hearts and minds to what was right there in front of them all along.

These real-life accounts suggest great ways to collect love-making data with (and about) our mate. Information is power, and learning about our partner is an important step in planning a successful journey to reignite the passion. The benefits and stim-ulation of open communication cannot be underestimated, espe-cially in the realm of sex and sexuality. The more we learn about our mate and the more we share with him, the greater the depths of intimacy and passion we can obtain.

Do we think we know all there is to know about our mate? We should think again. Sexuality is ever changing, and the topic is often difficult for people to discuss in any meaningful detail. The stories in this chapter are interesting, but they only scratch the surface of the deep and vast "passion pot of gold" that we can uncover if we journey to seek the passion *within him*.

LISA'S DESTINATIONS

The winters in Wisconsin are cold and harsh. By February, the gray sky is depressing and everyone is ready for spring. During these dark days, people such as Lisa and Paul plan a vacation to warmer climates. This sort of trip is motivation to shed those holiday pounds in preparation for the beach. Lisa was planning just such a vacation.

With time alone on the sand to look forward to, things were warming up in Lisa and Paul's bedroom. Just thinking about the warm sunny beaches and tropical nights caused a subtle change known as "vacation-anticipation sex." Lisa and Paul were work-ing out more in the bedroom as well as in the gym. Talking about and preparing for the impending trip stirred the embers enough to warm things up.

Lisa was shopping for sexy outfits and new swimsuits to wear at the fun, all-inclusive, adults-only resort she had found. For the first time in several years, they were going on vacation without the kids, and Lisa was thrilled to be trying something new. Her travel-agent friend had recommended the resort, saying it was like spring break for grown-ups. The travel brochure claimed it was the perfect place for a passion-filled second honeymoon.

They arrived at night around dinnertime and realized immediately what the travel agent meant about an adult's spring break. In the main dining room, a toga party was taking place that was unlike any toga party they had ever seen in college. There was a fair number of modest, Roman-style togas, but there was also a wide range of outfits, from the sexy to the bizarre.

When Paul and Lisa returned from dropping their luggage in their room, a conga line was making its way around the huge open-air dining room. Paul decided he was far too sober to deal with this environment and headed straight for the bar. Lisa, on the other hand, was thrilled and exhilarated. She thought about how the folks back home would be shocked to see where she was, not to mention what she was wearing. The look on Paul's face was one of "What have you gotten us into?"

The next morning, as they headed for the beach in their new swimsuits, they discovered they were overdressed. The majority of sunbathers walking by were wearing only their room key. Paul pointed out that he and Lisa were clearly at the clothing-optional end of the beach and immediately headed in the opposite direction. They discovered that there was in fact a nude beach and a prude beach at this resort. Paul expressed that he was proudly going to remain a prude.

Lisa's curiosity soon got the better of her, and within days she persuaded her husband to lie with her on the edge of the nude beach so that she could get a closer look. It was easy to convince him once she announced her plans to lie naked herself. Not believing she dared, and also feeling he needed to protect her, he followed. Lisa not only stripped down at the lounge chair but also walked over to the water to cool off and back again without wearing a stitch of clothing. This may not seem like a big deal to some, but for this conservative mother of three from the Midwest, the act was a turning point — she had gone from simply reading about these sorts of adventures to actually experiencing them.

Paul was not entirely convinced that Lisa was unaware ahead of time that the resort would feature such a large number of nudists. But despite feeling somewhat tricked, he sure liked the change in Lisa. She was more of the woman he remembered from their dating years. The mommy role had vanished, and she seemed so relaxed and free.

Paul had not yet reached this point. He was still decompressing from uptightville. The other guests at the resort were very helpful, though. They were extremely friendly and acted as if they were long-lost best friends, but Paul was still not comfortable with the nude beach. He would remove his trunks and dive straight into the waist-high water, keeping a good distance from most of the nudists. Nevertheless, even for Paul, it was impossible not to enjoy the freeing atmosphere or to watch the fun antics taking place at all hours of the day and night.

In a voyeuristic sense, the people-watching opportunities were incredible, not in a weird or dirty sort of way but rather in a natural "the human body is beautiful in all its shapes and sizes" sort of way. Lisa and Paul saw it all. They did not even know that the body could be pierced in some of those places or that people could have such extraordinary anatomical differences! And the free displays of affection were shocking at times, yet not shocking at all. The resort seemed such a natural environment, so relaxing and freeing. No uptight dress codes. No uptight anything. This was simply an opportunity to be really present with one's mate and nothing else — no deadlines, curfews, parental responsibilities, cares, or expectations.

In this environment Paul and Lisa found it nearly impossible not to cut loose and enjoy themselves. The ambience of the resort was very stimulating — just the kind of passion quest the couple needed. Their impressions of what they saw or guessed might be going on around them acted as stimulants in the bedroom. Their "vacation-sex high" reached an even higher level — one that they had never imagined possible.

It was especially fun at night to watch other couples and groups, trying to imagine what they were doing or going to do, and what they were into and what they were not. The conversations were even better. Paul and Lisa were surprised at the things people told them in the anonymous environment of the vacation resort. The couple met so many different people from all walks of life and from all over the world — honeymooners, baby boomers, Italian swingers, German bikers, and Canadian doctors.

One night, Lisa encouraged Paul to check out the pool bar and Jacuzzi with her. There was always a lot of music and laughter emanating from that area of the resort, especially late at night. As they sat cuddled in a lounge chair a short distance away from the crowded spa waters, Lisa devised a guessing game with her husband. What are they into, what do they want, who are they with, and who will they leave with? It was fun for Lisa to imagine what was going on under the bubbly waters, and she got an inkling at times watching the faces of the people as they talked and laughed. Sometimes she was tipped off by a knowing glance or an appreciative sigh. Sometimes it was an unmistakable display of serious affection. In any case, it was all quite an aphrodisiac.

Paul and Lisa found themselves running back to their hotel room to make love many times throughout the day and night. They were having sex more frequently than they had during their honeymoon nearly a decade and a half ago. They already recognized the advantage of "getting away from it all," but this experience went beyond that. This was the warm sun and tropical fruity drinks, the friendly people, the freeing environment of the nude beach, the romantic sunsets, and the opportunity to dress up and go out on "dates" with one's mate to theme parties each evening. It was all this and more, allowing for a much-needed break to nurture the passion in their relationship.

Most noteworthy of their discoveries that week was what Lisa learned about her mate. Sure, Paul was uptight at first, but after he decompressed, the environment allowed Lisa to observe her husband in a new and different light. Watching him reacting to what he saw was as interesting to Lisa as the goings-on themselves.

Lisa was realizing that she was getting a unique opportunity to rediscover what Paul did and did not find appealing. Her husband's reactions and comments were telling, even in the way he observed how the women dressed and flirted. Lisa said she always felt she knew Paul inside and out, but not until they found themselves in this relaxed, socially stimulating environment did she realize the ways in which he had grown and the ways in which his tastes had subtly changed through the years.

This newfound information was an advantage to Lisa in many ways. She was paying attention to her husband and viewing him in a way she rarely did at home. By breaking out of the routine and away from the expected, Lisa was seeing Paul not just in his everyday roles as spouse, father, and breadwinner but also as a sexual being with distinct needs, desires, and passions.

In reexamining her view of her mate and placing him in a different light, Lisa was able to step outside the familiar and rediscover the passion within him — the passion that made her blood boil in those heated early days of their relationship. This was just the beginning of Lisa's journey. The quest for knowledge was just starting, and there was so much more to learn about her mate.

The vacation week flew by, and as Paul and Lisa left for home, the couple realized they would likely come back to this resort someday. The days and weeks that followed their return were heated from the memories of the passion-filled escape they had experienced. And thus the cycle began: Lisa and Paul found a route to a never-ending passion quest by seeking out second-honeymoon locations for their annual sun pilgrimage. The anticipation of the vacation to come, the cutting loose once there, and then the reliving of the fun in their memories once they returned home provided a continual source of heat to keep the passion flame burning brightly — for a while.

A Stop at the Next Port

Lisa was not ashamed of where they went on vacation and certainly was not ashamed of anything they did. They were married, and Lisa's viewpoint was that passion was a gift from God that she and Paul were meant to share and enjoy to the fullest. She was not going to pretend that she felt any other way, but unfortunately she was finding that some of her colleagues had strange notions about nudity and adult resorts. They assumed the worst and conjured up all sorts of images of the taboo, especially in the conservative community in which she lived.

So after that first vacation to an all-inclusive adults-only resort, Lisa learned to keep her mouth shut about what she did on vacation. She found that some people tended to think in extremes and could condemn them for their actions. Lisa thought that maybe these people lived such uptight and unhappy lives that they had to believe everyone else was having boring married sex or, if they were not, must be doing something forbidden.

Lisa loved her vacation away, though, and she came home relaxed and feeling passionately in love. After that first tropical vacation alone with Paul, she vowed to find a way to escape annually. The very next year, however, they decided to go with friends to Hawaii instead. The trip was fun and relaxing, but it did not allow for the passionate freedom they felt when they were alone together. Having friends on vacation took away the opportunity to have intimate time with just one's mate. The guys would go off golfing, and the gals would shop or sunbathe. The year prior, without friends from home around, Lisa and Paul spent more time in intimate conversation with each other, and even though they were not often technically alone in such a party environment, the atmosphere was more conducive to passion.

As a result, the following year they were drawn back to the resort — to their tropical getaway filled with friendly partyers and "interesting" scenery. The trip was again eye-opening, with so much to learn from the antics of others. For Lisa, this next vacation was an education on how to play safely and an opportunity to take a new look at her mate.

On the beach early one day, Lisa met a couple, and after talking with them for some time, she invited them to join her and Paul in the dining room that evening. While getting ready in their room, Paul commented on how attractive the couple was and asked Lisa if she agreed. Soon the conversation turned sexual, with Paul asking Lisa if she would really ever want to swing if the right couple came along. Lisa said that she had been intrigued by the idea ever since that chance encounter in Las Vegas and thought that yes, she might be interested under the right circumstances.

Paul and Lisa then began a conversation about what exactly the right circumstances would be and what their limitations were. Paul insisted that oral sex would be out of the question and that only intercourse with condoms would be acceptable. The discussion eventually became heated and not in a good way. Finally, as Paul and Lisa were leaving their hotel room, they agreed that they had a great deal too many rules about what they should and should not do, and there was too much room for error because these rules were not concrete. Therefore, they decided the whole idea was too fraught with potential hazards and should be avoided for now.

Lisa and Paul found themselves in a different situation later that evening. After dinner, the couple they dined with suggested they all head down to the beach. With another bottle of wine in hand, they did just that. The other couple, whom we will call Brad and Pamela, decided to skinny-dip in the wading pool near the beach. Paul and Lisa were soon in the pool as well. After some playing around in the water, Brad pulled Pamela out of the pool, laid her down on some beach towels, and started kissing her, among other things. Much to Lisa's surprise, Paul followed suit, and soon they were also in the throes of passion, lying very near the other couple. It was a huge turn-on for Lisa to hear Brad and Pamela so close by, breathing heavily and moaning. She turned her head just enough so that she could see them clearly. It was like having a live porn movie right in front of them while they made love.

Lisa noticed Pamela watching Paul. Pamela whispered to Lisa that she was impressed and then encouraged Paul with some very nasty talk. Soon, Brad and Pamela were finished, and Paul and Lisa continued while the other couple watched. Paul lasted for what seemed like an eternity while Pamela masturbated watching them and especially watching Paul. It was amazing to Lisa to see this woman so turned on by Paul and by what he was doing to his wife. It was a unique opportunity. Lisa was seeing her husband reflected in this woman's eyes, and she loved what she saw.

Lisa saw Paul as if she were seeing him again for the first time and has replayed the experience in her mind many times since that night. For now, Lisa told me, these memories are more than enough. She does not feel the need to cross the line and journey into the land of swingers. She has *no* desire to share her mate with anyone.

Maybe swinging works for some people. Maybe it is a viable solution to boredom in the marital bed or maybe it is a recipe for disaster. It depends on the individuals involved and what makes sense for their relationship. At one point, Lisa had not been sure if her curiosity would overcome her caution. She is now no longer uncertain. She has learned all she needs to know. For Lisa and Paul's relationship, simple curiosity is not enough. Swinging simply does not feel right.

The couple spent their last night alone in what they came to feel was paradise. They walked the beach hand in hand and made love by moonlight. Lisa was thrilled to have her husband all to herself and hoped that would be the case for years to come.

COURTNEY'S EXPLORATIONS

In chapter 8, we discussed Courtney, the stay-at-home mother of three whose husband, Jim, was very demanding sexually. Although they had sex several times a week, making love did not come easy for them anymore. They had to work at creating excitement. They had sought out new and different locations to have sex and had tried a few three-ways with other women, but they still felt there was little left to explore. The question we were left with was, just what would Courtney and Jim try in order to improve their sex life this time?

Courtney had long fantasized about unconventional methods to spice things up in her marriage. She and her husband had made some of these fantasies a reality. Their wild explorations had involved some emotional risk, but Courtney had not yet shied away from the path less taken. She wanted to have a male guest in their bed this time. Jim was uncomfortable with the idea, but Courtney felt this next step was only fair. Where would this debate take them? Courtney would eventually discover a lot about her husband and the strength of their relationship when she headed down the path to further explore the wild side.

Courtney was pushing the issue with Jim, but he was not budging. Homophobic issues aside, he did not feel he could bear seeing Courtney in the throes of passion with another man. After several attempts to persuade him and much arguing, Courtney was convinced by her girlfriends to give it a rest. Nothing good ever came from pushing a spouse into something he did not want any part of.

Courtney realized that she was perhaps making too much of the issue. Sure, she wanted to even the score, so to speak, by having her chance with a man joining her and her husband, but it certainly would not be any fun if Jim was uncomfortable with it. Plus, the issue was not that she really cared that much about having a three-way with a man but rather that she was bored with the same old routine — wiping the damn kitchen counter off fifty times a day, doing laundry, dropping the kids off here and picking them up there, not to mention the missionary-position "quickies" with Jim before they both collapsed at night. Courtney was tired of constantly performing for everyone. She was the perfect little Stepford wife, always doing what hubby asked of her, always taking good care of her husband and the children, and always saying yes whenever anyone asked for help. Rarely did she do anything for herself.

She had become the bored housewife she swore she would never be. This was not because she had nothing to do but rather because she lacked anything exciting to do. There was no stimulation in her daily existence. The question was where to go now for some excitement, and not just sexually. All her major life decisions were behind her: career, marriage, family, and children. What was there to look forward to that was new and exciting?

Courtney was going to find a way to spice things up. She was not about to give up without a fight. She was determined to go on a passion quest to find what was missing, crank up the heat, and keep the fires burning brightly for years to come.

The Journey for the Missing Passion Continues

Courtney had been reading up on hot-spot clubs and conventions for adults. She convinced Jim to check out a sexy nightclub that was actually not far away. Courtney was able to accomplish this by promising that if the club was not fun, she would go with her husband to an exotic dancers' club instead. She even vowed to put a few dollars in the G-string of the woman of his choice, or encourage him to do so himself. This did the trick.

The nightclub was filled with well-dressed patrons, and the sound system was extremely loud. Jim did not usually care to dance, so Courtney was set loose to find her own dance partner while Jim stood nearby. He loved to watch his wife dance, and Courtney loved to perform for him. It was arousing for both of them. This did not work at home, though, because with the children nearby, the atmosphere was simply not conducive. No, it had to be when they were dressed up and at a club or large party where the ambience was right.

This club was just what they needed. Courtney asked a couple dancing nearby if she could join them. She danced a set or two and then went to have a drink with her husband, but he ushered her out to the valet and quickly home to make love. Just that little bit of outside stimulation made a huge difference for them that night — something that dinner and a movie with friends could never do.

Another night at the same club brought about a unique opportunity. Jim was at the bar ordering drinks while Courtney danced alone on the edge of the large dance floor. She noticed a couple watching her and smiled at them. Sometime later in the evening she saw the same couple on the dance floor nearby and asked if she could join them. They smiled and nodded. Courtney was very attracted to the man, and come to think of it, the woman was appealing also. Courtney worked her best dance moves and flirted with them shamelessly.

Off the dance floor, Jim questioned her. What was she up to and where did she see it heading? She admitted to her husband that they had invited her — just her — back to their hotel room nearby. Jim thought the whole idea was crazy, since she did not know this couple at all. It was not safe to go off with them alone.

He did agree, however, to meet them for dinner the next night. Dinner was fun. The couple was in town for several days visiting family. They seemed normal, and Jim relaxed. But when he was away from the table, the couple again asked Courtney if she would join them alone, without her husband.

Courtney was extremely tempted. In her mind, this kind of experience would even the score. She had allowed Jim, on two occasions no less, to have a three-way with another woman. He wanted no part of inviting a man into their bedroom, so this was her opportunity to experience something similar without putting Jim in an awkward position. The question was, by asking Jim to let her go with this couple alone, would she be putting him in just as awkward a position? Would he really be willing to allow Courtney this experience without repercussions?

Courtney soon got an answer to her questions. It was as if the moon and stars were aligning to make it happen. Their cell phone rang, and the babysitter needed them to come home. Jim suggested to Courtney that she stay and have fun, and the other couple offered to drive her home later. Courtney walked Jim to the door of the restaurant and asked if he realized what he was doing. Was he really agreeing to let her "mess around" with this couple by herself? The answer was yes, he was going to give her this gift, as he called it. He recognized how much she wanted to try something new, and frankly he was tired of her restlessness.

Courtney did not question him but immediately jumped at the chance. She soon left with the couple to their hotel room. The experience proved to be amazing for Courtney. She felt like a queen with two sex slaves at her disposal. They spoiled her with their attentions. Never had she imagined what it would be like to be the visitor in a three-way with a couple. They both fed off her body. She was unsure if they were enjoying themselves as much as she was, but she found she did not really care either.

They were talking to each other as if she could not hear them or as if she were only there in body. The woman said such things to her mate as, "Look at her breasts. They are so beautiful." And he said, "My God, how reactive she is when I touch her with my tongue right here." This did not make her feel like a sex toy but rather like royalty. It was surreal.

The Travel Fares Increase

Returning to reality was difficult the next day, especially since Jim was acting so strange. Actually, Courtney was unsure if he was really acting strange or if she was projecting. She felt as if her nerve endings were still on fire and actually felt raw. In bed that next night, Jim wanted to know all the details about what had happened. Courtney was unsure if this was such a good idea. She was still incredibly turned on by it all and did not want to risk spoiling the mood by saying something that would upset Jim. Should she tell him how amazing it was or tone it down a little?

She ended up confessing everything, and they had fabulous sex that night. However, Courtney immediately noticed a change in Jim. He seemed uncomfortable and almost insecure. It was going to take work to repair the unspoken damage that had occurred. Unfortunately, Courtney was completely unsure as to what the issue or problem was. Was he testing her that night and did not really think she would go through with it? Was he upset that she enjoyed it? Did it somehow make him feel insecure about their relationship? He would not shed any light on the situation. In fact, he insisted that nothing was wrong.

But something was wrong. Jim did not seem to trust her anymore. He would show up at home or the gym when he was not expected. He started saying "I love you" all the time, which would have been a good thing if it did not come across as forced and unnatural. He would call to check up on her at strange times of the day or night, whether he was in town or not. Courtney felt as if she had an overdue bill to pay. The ledger was not balanced between them — Jim had the advantage and Courtney was going to have to fight to catch up. Again, this did not seem fair. Why weren't they even?

Courtney was never one to keep her mouth shut about anything. She usually told her closest friends all her secrets, and this mess was no exception. The quest for passion, she explained, was actually a success. Jim and Courtney were certainly having spicier sex, but the weirdness outside the bedroom had to stop. The group concluded that although the situation did not seem fair, Courtney was going to have to pay her dues if she really cared about the relationship.

Courtney was not going to take responsibility for Jim's reactions, but she was easily convinced by her close girlfriend to take responsibility for *her own actions.* If she did not like what she got in response to her wild escapades, then maybe she needed to try something else. If she was determined to accept the bad in order to keep the good, then she had to acknowledge that he was simply not capable of dealing with such sexual explorations as well as she could.

Courtney had to be reminded that it was not all that long ago when she and Jim had experienced that first three-way with a woman. After that event, *Courtney* was the one who had trouble dealing with the experience. She simply could not sort out the dichotomy of her emotions at the time. She had felt weird about how much she had enjoyed it while at the same time feeling a little insecure about her relationship. Reflecting on this helped Courtney put Jim's reactions into proper perspective.

She needed to cut her husband a little slack. After all, he did not even get to participate in the encounter. He had been left out entirely.

Time, they say, heals all wounds, and Courtney certainly hoped this would be the case. She had quickly gotten over her struggle with their first three-way, so perhaps Jim would soon be okay with what had happened. She was not one to simply wait things out, though. Instead, Courtney was determined to put full effort into helping the relationship heal and at the same time not allow their marriage to ever detour again from their passion-seeking journey for two.

Exploring the Exotic Together

Courtney's first effort to patch things up was to surprise Jim with a trip to an exotic dance club. He had requested such an evening out on previous occasions, and she knew how much he enjoyed seeing women dance. Courtney herself was not put out by the idea. She felt the human body was beautiful, and a woman's curves and sex appeal were no exception. She knew how soft and inviting a woman could be, and although she was happy with her heterosexual lifestyle, she could visually (and even physically) appreciate a woman from time to time.

Courtney knew this would be a sexy and, more important, a safe way to spice up the relationship. She had read that it was no longer uncommon for women to attend such clubs and even get into the fun, offering the dancers some bills in their garters. In addition, Courtney thought this would be a great opportunity to watch her husband and collect some data. Bare minimum, she might pick up some dance moves for the bedroom.

Putting more effort into pleasing him, and actually taking note of *his* preferences and attempting to fulfill *his* fantasies, sets the wheels in motion for having the favors returned.

Although dark and smoky, the club was a top-notch establishment. In fact, the large cover charge likely kept out some questionable patrons. The furnishings and decorations appeared to be of high quality and the sound system was great. Courtney was sure this place was a rarity in its class of clubs. More important, the dancers were not disappointing. There were a surprising number of beautiful women, and all of them had great bodies.

There were low, circular tables with comfy cushioned chairs around them. There were girls everywhere. A number of dancers were giving table dances with patrons sitting a few feet away, ogling them with their eyes. The dance on the main stage was impressive, with almost acrobatic moves taking place in time to the music. As their eyes slowly adjusted, Jim and Courtney sat down at a table in the middle of the high-ceilinged room.

Courtney watched Jim and asked him to tell her when he saw something he liked. They discussed the dancers at length, and Courtney took note of what her husband seemed most interested in. This was not just a lesson in body shape and hair color but also in sexy bedroom attire and most significantly in movement. The dancers had all the sexy maneuvers down pat in many and varied styles. It was not only educational but extremely sensual to watch.

Courtney thought the men were interesting to watch as well. Their reactions and flirtations with the dancers were at times amusing, at times sexy, and at times annoying. Most interesting, though, was the way her own husband was responding. She found it especially fascinating to watch him from a distance as she was returning from the bathroom.

On one of these trips to the powder room, she paid a dancer to give Jim a lap dance. When he was told by the dancer that his wife had bought him a dance, he looked up to find Courtney, but she quickly ducked behind a large support beam. She then peeked out while the woman danced for her husband. It was both stimulating and agitating to watch him become mesmerized by the dancer.

Courtney returned to the table to find that Jim had paid the dancer to now dance for her. The dancer kept throwing her long brown hair onto Courtney and touching Courtney in what appeared to be a need to keep her balance in her platform heels. When the song ended, the dancer sat down at their table and started making small talk. For a rare moment, Courtney was speechless. She found herself turned on by the dancer but even more so by her husband and the looks they gave each other as the woman danced.

The evening was a huge success in Courtney's eyes. She had found a stimulating adventure in their passion-seeking journey. For weeks afterward, they talked about the dancers during love-making. Courtney had picked up a few dance pointers that worked both in and out of bed. She also had been clued in to a few outfits that Jim had found appealing. One night, Courtney tried out a baby-doll nightie and donned a long wig similar to that worn by one of the dancers. Another night, she expanded on a different dancer's leopard motif by wearing an actual cat costume.

Her efforts were well received by Jim, and he in turn showed his appreciation. By putting more effort into pleasing him, and actually taking note of *his* preferences and attempting to fulfill *his* fantasies, Courtney set the wheels in motion for having the favors returned. With Courtney's example to follow, he became bolder himself and began to take notice of her ever-changing needs.

To *truly* travel together is to reap the greatest rewards.

Courtney loved sharing wild explorations with her husband. When she had gone off by herself with the other couple, she had experienced negative long-term effects in her relationship with Jim. Recognizing this was important for Courtney in a number of ways. She was looking at her husband in a new light. She was seeing his role in her expeditions as one of utmost importance. It was not about getting something for herself but about the heights they could attain together.

Learning to find the new in the old without constantly needing to venture into wild explorations was now a lifetime goal for Courtney and Jim's love affair. This was not the easiest route to take. Sometimes wild explorations still pulled them down risky paths, but they always recognized the ultimate goal. To *truly* travel together is to reap the greatest rewards.

A New Look at Our Old Mate — Travel Data and Research

Both Lisa and Courtney learned a lot about their mate when they really paid attention — or in some cases when they were put in positions where they could not help but notice. Their stories were not included in this book to provide mere voyeuristic entertainment but rather to teach us some important lessons about how to (and how maybe not to) take a new look and rediscover the passion within *him*. The route we choose in order to accomplish this will be our own.

Before we set out with our mate on passionate explorations — whether these expeditions are wild or tame — we will benefit greatly from conducting research and gathering data about him. In planning any successful journey, we must learn more about our partner and share more with him in order to reach greater depths of intimacy and passion. So if our goal is to reignite the passion in our long-term relationship or even just keep the journey moving forward, we must take a *new* look at our old mate and rediscover what is right there in front of us.

> Information is power, and gathering it is an important step in planning a successful journey seeking passion with our mate.

To be intimately involved with someone requires that before we depart on any quest for passion, we must do the research, whether we have traveled with the person before or not. We must scope out destinations, draw up an itinerary, and plan the best routes to take on this unique passion journey. The research has to be conducted with (and about) our travel companion. Specifically, we have to recognize and understand our partner, including his *current* limitations, preferences, and desires. We cannot expect to have a successful journey if we plan the trip without him in mind, or plan it based on outdated information.

Of course, our own needs and desires are equally as important and must be recognized. The point is that we are not taking this passion quest alone. Just as we learned in kindergarten, if we want to play well with others, we have to consider what games they want to play and take turns.

Therefore our passion quest for two requires that we take continuing-education courses. No matter how well-read we are or how practiced we are in the areas of sexual technique, there is always more to learn. We can use magazines, books, movies, Web sites, and chat rooms to collect data to incorporate into our lovemaking journeys. In planning the itinerary, we should review these materials with our mate and learn what interests him, as well as share with him what looks interesting to us. Then we can make a date to visit the agreed upon destinations. Sometimes, though, we may need to take turns. We must keep an open mind and consider stopovers that we do not think we are really interested in. We may end up being surprised with the experience and find that it is a great idea after all. As long as we put some effort into planning the itinerary ahead of time — with his input or at least with him in mind — we have a great chance of finding passion along the way.

When reassessing what appeals to our mate — and most important in *sharing* these desires with him — we might try bringing home the latest issues of *Playboy* or some other such "skin" magazine. We can even use our Victoria's Secret catalogs, showing him which women and outfits we think are appealing and asking him which ones he likes and why. Reading erotica together to determine which stories appeal to him is also an effective method. We should try these suggestions even if we feel we already know his tastes. Things change as we grow and mature. We may be surprised. Even just the act of looking through the material and showing interest in him can make a difference; at the very least it can provide momentary mood enhancement and create some intimacy. This sort of research will bring us closer to our mate, and eventually he will feel as if he is able to open up to us more and really share his desires and fantasies.

Examining Explicit Travel Brochures — A Note About Visual Stimulation Research

One day a younger friend of mine was complaining to me about her husband. The couple had been married only a short time, and she could not understand why he wanted or needed to have nude magazines, pornographic movies, or any materials of the sort. She felt as if he should be completely happy with looking at just her body — why did he need more? She had gotten upset with him and was going to insist he get rid of the materials. I told her that maybe he would be okay with that and would do as she wished. Then again, she might end up forcing him to go underground with his materials. So I asked her if there was any way she would be able to accept this about him and find methods to incorporate such materials into their intimate relationship. Would she rather share this with him or possibly have him go behind her back?

Passion Seekers agree that how threatening such materials are is in direct correlation to how secure one feels about one's relationship and about oneself. I reassured my newlywed friend that her husband's interests were certainly not uncommon. Men tend to enjoy visual stimulation. We can either accept this or struggle against it. I, for one, think that to fight this inclination is a losing battle. If we feel good about ourselves and remember that our mate picked us above all others, then we should not be threatened by such materials. It is far more productive to embrace and share in our partner's interests. We may even enjoy these pursuits ourselves.

> The benefits and stimulation of open communication cannot be underestimated, especially in the realm of sex and sexuality.

If in the past we have continually fought against such visual stimulation, we will now face difficulty in getting our partner to open up about his interests. He will fear reprisal and worry about hurting us, especially if he has previously been beaten down on the subject. Some men are going to be extremely gun-shy about discussing or looking at other beautiful women with their mate, let alone talking explicitly about sex, particularly if their mate has already complained about visual stimulation — or

worse, has been angry about it. Only time and patience (and perhaps the implementation of some of the ideas set out below) will
remedy the situation.

Researching a Passion Quest Can Be as Fun as the Quest Itself

> The more we learn about him and the more we share with him,
> the greater the depths of intimacy and passion we will achieve.

For those who truly wish to appreciate, understand, and
share in the depths of their mate's sexuality, and in the process
obtain deeper and more meaningful levels of intimacy, placing
data-collection techniques high on the list of priorities is a must.
Some of these techniques may make perfect sense for our relationship, and some may be out of the question. Whatever our situation, we must never sit back contentedly with the belief that
we know all there is to know about our mate and all there is to
know about seeking passion.

The opportunities and possibilities for doing research with
and about our mate are endless. One idea is to try sitting down at
the computer *together.* Instead of surfing the Web alone, we can
share the time with our mate, searching for fun sites or going
into chat rooms. Chatting with an online stranger can be hilari-
ous, as we try to guess whether the person is male or female.
Both partners might formulate questions or queries together and
see what replies they get back. There are some wild, fun, and
kinky sites out there. Who knows what we will find or *what we
might learn about our mate* if we share this time with him.

Another fun idea is to go to the bookstore with our partner
and browse the sex-help section for interesting titles. The
shelves are full of guidebooks, including those on wild positions,

Kama Sutra, sexy talk, erotic stories, and so much more. This is a very popular section of any bookstore and can be fun and amusing to search through with our mate. We may find something that appeals to each partner. If each person selects a book (or one book to share), both partners can then read the book and mark it up to create their own "bedroom-technique wish list." This list (or the places we mark in the book) should focus on what we would like to try or do more often. This way we can share our desires in a nonthreatening, less embarrassing way — and even have diagrams to help. Such research about (and with) our mate is invaluable to any quest for passion.

There is, of course, the simple technique of looking at magazines and reading erotica together. This will not only open up the spectrum of bedroom possibilities but also provide a unique opportunity to rediscover what is and is not turning our mate on. Any information we gather about our mate is powerful, not just to ensure that we do not hit a dead end in our passion quest but ultimately to make certain we are placing priority on our travel mate's needs as well as our own.

Just having our mate read us an erotic story or create one to share with us will tell us a lot about what he finds arousing. Which story did he choose to read to us? What elements of the story could we incorporate into our sexual encounters with him? Or we can play the Passion Seekers' Party Game set out in chapter 10 and really listen to his answers. We might just learn a thing or two.

Although trying something new might end up being a passion quest itself, the venturing forth is also a great way to reacquaint ourselves with our mate and collect data to continue on a successful and exciting journey. Both Lisa and Courtney learned a lot about their mate and saw him in a new light when they journeyed into unknown lands. The "something new" does not have to be an exotic or wild exploration. It can be any different experience for us to share with our mate. We might go camping or hiking, take dancing lessons, try new sporting adventures as Carla and John did — anything new to share alone with our mate. We will see him in a different light, out of his regular roles and possibly out of his comfort zone. This new perspective has helped some to reignite the passion.

The following is a brief summary of ideas that others have used successfully in researching their travel partner. We recognize that communication is vital in all aspects of our long-term relationship and that discussion does not have to be a chore. These simple and sexy ideas are fun ways to open up the lines of communication and discover something new about our old mate.

Get Reacquainted with Your Travel Partner — Passion Seekers' Research Ideas

- Visit the bookstore together and create a "bedroom-technique wish list."
- Do Internet research. Surf the Web with your mate and share "chats."
- Review "skin" magazines together and discuss what each of you finds sexy.
- Share sexy movies — let him select.
- Have your mate tell you an erotic story or have him select one to read to you.
- Try something new and exciting together, such as dance lessons, scuba diving, camping, etc.
- Visit somewhere new — a nude beach, an adults-only resort, a nightclub, etc.
- Play the Passion Seekers' Party Game (chapter 10).
- Just spend time alone together (not at the movies or in front of the TV).

The information we acquire by paying attention to what appeals to our mate will pay off big both in the bedroom and out. Even if we have been with our partner for a long time, if we really pay attention, we will discover new and untapped passions within him — and within ourselves. We may realize that we have only scratched the surface, but if we dig a little deeper, we may uncover treasures that we never imagined.

CHAPTER TEN

THE PASSION SEEKERS' CLUB

The Passion Seekers' Club is the ultimate excuse for a girls' night out. In this chapter I share the titillating ideas and secrets of the passion quest support group and how it evolved into the Passion Seekers' Club — a group that helps us to have healthier relationships with our mate and fills our life with "that feels great!" intimacy. A little bit of focus on our sexual selves and time spent confiding and sharing with our friends makes a dramatic difference in the quest to find the missing passion — and to keep it alive.

The many responses and e-mails I have received from my Web site, PassionSeekers.com, have alerted me to the nearly desperate need to put some focus and priority on passion and intimacy in our life. So many relationships suffer from sexual mediocrity and often neglect. The problem permeates all aspects of our existence, and some do not even recognize the problem.

Not counting sarcastic comments or jokes, when was the last time we talked to our friends about our sex life? It has probably been a long time. When we were single, many of us talked to our friends about sex. Somehow, though, since we got married, sex seems to have become a very rare topic. We talk about everything else in great detail and dole out ample suggestions and advice. Why don't we put a little focus on this vital topic?

Our moms probably shared and learned a lot over coffee at the neighbor's kitchen table. Unlike our moms or grandmothers, who were often around the neighborhood all day, we really have to work at simply getting together with friends. We are all juggling so many different roles and responsibilities. Our jobs and our kids consume us. If we do not consciously make the time and put the effort into continually seeking passion with our mate, the romance will slip away and cease to exist in our lives. We need to take a lesson from our moms or grandmothers and get together with our friends to really talk. A support group can make a huge difference in these efforts.

I had been recording real-life dramas about couples pursuing passion for some time before the birth of the Passion Seekers — that fateful night when my friends and I challenged one another to a passion quest. Since that first meeting, the idea of a Passion Seekers' Club took hold and rapidly grew in intensity. Once people realize what is missing in their life or, rather, what they are missing out on, they all want to become Passion Seekers. Life is just too short to be grinding away without the depth of pleasure and intimacy we can attain in our long-term relationship when we set our mind to it.

Our passion quest support group began by accident. Too many martinis and a few confessions later, we discovered the perfect excuse for a regular girls' night out. This experience evolved into the Passion Seekers. Sometimes we combine our Passion Seekers' discussions with other activities, such as scrap-booking or attending one of those parties where a representative is trying to sell us baskets, jewelry, or the latest trendy food prod-ucts. Whether we have talked over cocktails or coffee, we all agree that the support and suggestions we have gotten, the top-ics we've discussed, and most of all the fun we have had have made a dramatic difference in our relationship with our mate, in our friendships, and in our attitude toward sex and intimacy.

We share problems, desires, ideas, and solutions. Passion Seekers learn from one another and are in turn inspired to try something different and report back with the results. Tip sharing is great fun and has caused some lively discussions. We also use the passion quest suggestion bowl, which requires that we each contribute to the pot with written tips or suggestions on small sheets of paper. Some of my friends bring typed tips so no one can identify their handwriting. Sharing these ideas results in some wild discussions. For example, one tip was to give "mini–blow jobs" to different parts of our mate's body such as to his fingers, toes, and earlobes. The comments flew about that one. The key is to learn from one another and use that knowl-edge to stimulate our creativity at home.

These informal meetings, sometimes happening sponta-neously over cocktails at the country club, were the beginnings of more formal support groups and have even led to workshops. Whatever the setting, the goal is to positively support one another in our long-term relationship quest. Fun and games pro-vide subtle stimulation and remind us that we must feed the pas-sion in our relationship if we do not wish it to slowly starve to death.

When we share with other women, we discover there is

nothing wrong with us. We find answers to questions we did not know to ask, and we are inspired to put more effort into making love, thus finding more pleasure and joy in our marriage or long-term relationship. The night that my friends and I opened up to one another for the very first time, every one of our mates got laid when we got home. Just a little bit of focus on our sexual selves, and the intimacy and pleasure we long for, caused us to not just have sex but have it *enthusiastically.*

Our innate sexual desires and needs are begging to be met. We have to pay attention to them and recognize the important role they play in our relationship. We have to place a priority on our quest for passion. This is the goal of the support group. So even if we are meeting with our sister or our closest friend, chatting online, or attending a regular club, we must find a place in our life for the fun and intimacy of sharing. We need to give ourselves permission to seek passion because our involvement will ultimately bring huge benefits to our marriage.

We are reminded that we must continually feed the passion in our relationship if we do not wish it to slowly starve to death.

The topic of conversation at our meetings has varied from discussing how we "often do not feel like it," to how to talk dirty and not feel silly about it, to unusual locations for lovemaking, to sexual dysfunction, to you name it. Other than our mate, whom do we really talk to about sex? Most of us would sooner choke than discuss the topic with our mothers or, for that matter, our doctors. Even the input of well-meaning therapists is limited by professional protocol and personal experience. The real education comes from hearing about the successes and failures in real-life relationships. We can talk to our friends and form a Passion Seekers' group. If our peers do not have a suggestion or idea, they can at least listen and perhaps help us sort out what is right for our relationship.

> *The Passion Seekers' Motto:* Seeking the passion in our relationship will send us on the road to a happier, healthier, and more relaxed self. We must enjoy ourselves while we still can and our relationship while we still have it!

PASSION SEEKERS' PARTY IDEAS

What we do at our Passion Seekers' meetings and parties is not about *working* on anything; it is about fun and about stimulating the passion flame in our relationship. Passion Seekers' activities can take place with just an intimate group of friends, as after-dinner entertainment at a couples' dinner party, or with a group of strangers in a workshop setting. Some of these activities have occurred in the wee hours of a large party, when only the die-hard party guests remained. Whatever the gathering, the goal is to have entertaining and stimulating conversations that motivate us to seek passion for the health of our marriage. The following list summarizes the focus of this chapter, which is to have fun with the topic of passion and, in the process, enrich our most important long-term relationship.

Passion Seekers' Party Ideas

- Exchanging sexy books, CDs, and movies
- Using a passion quest suggestion bowl — collecting ideas and tips for discussion
- Holding a Passion Seekers' Book Club (or Passion Methodology Book Club) meeting
- Forming a "sex in the mass media" discussion group

- Taking a field trip to the local adult bookstore
- Hosting a "white-elephant sex toy" gift exchange
- Completing and sharing Passion Seekers' anonymous surveys (found on PassionSeekers.com under "Passion Poll")
- Playing the Passion Seekers' Party Game outlined in this chapter

Whether we invite "just the girls" or several couples over to our home, we can ask everyone to bring a passion-enhancing sexy book or movie to exchange. Books should have the sexy parts marked accordingly. The items should be labeled with the person's name (so they can eventually be returned) and then placed in a box by the front door. When each person or couple leaves for the evening, they will select something from the box to take home and enjoy with their mate.

The passion quest suggestion bowl mentioned earlier is a fun addition to any adult get-together. We can place a passion pot on the refreshment table with a sign asking everyone to write down on a piece of paper a passion-enhancing idea, tip, product recommendation, or other sexy suggestion. Then the participants put the slips of paper into the pot. Later in the evening, the hostess will draw the slips out and read them off — no one will know who wrote what! As an alternative, after the pot is filled up, we can place it at the front door with a sign suggesting that each person draw a slip out of the bowl to take home. Either way, we are potentially enhancing the passion in a few of our guests' beds later that night!

The Passion Seekers' Book Club is another mood-enhancing activity to share with friends. In advance of the meeting, we assign a sexy or romantic novel for the group to read, then set a date for discussion. Topics may include the building of passion in the book, how the author creates mood, or how a particular scene in the book can be used to reignite the passion in our own lives. The key is to relax, have a few cocktails, and share some ideas and tips to spice things up at home.

A different twist on the book club is the Passion Methodology Book Club, in which members share and discuss sex-technique or sex-help books. To get started, I have listed a few favorite sex-technique books in the resources section at the back of this book. Before the meeting, we should try some of the selected book's suggestions in our own bed. At the gathering, the hostess will read a few book-review notes that she has prepared in advance to get the discussion going, and then we will talk, share, and laugh about what worked and what did not. Some of the positions and techniques in these books may be comical, but some turn out to be earth-shattering discoveries.

Another tip-sharing technique is the "sex in the mass media" discussion group. Each meeting requires that the members bring a magazine, newspaper, or Internet article on either a chosen or an assigned sex topic. Attendees summarize their article for the group, and the subject is opened for discussion. Whether we learn something new, are inspired to step out of our routine, or just have a fun time debating the merits of the articles, the evening will be fun and motivating in our quest for passion.

An active trading ring of Passion Seekers' movie, music, and book picks is also recommended. We can borrow our friends' romantic or even trashy novels and share an occasional tech-nique video, sexy movie, or passion-inducing CD. This is a great way to not only try out a book, movie, or CD before buying it but also find out what others recommend. When I first asked my friends to share their favorite items, I was surprised to discover that, other than some music CDs, few of them had any sugges-tions. Do we really spend such little time on mood-enhancing media, or are there just so few really excellent sexy movies and books out there? I have to believe that we are simply not seeking out such sources. This is a shame because reading books and watching movies are quick ways to enhance our mood and put us in the passion quest frame of mind.

A good way for us to use a sexy novel or romance book is the following: When we reach a part of the novel where things get hot, we should not wait to finish the chapter or the book. Instead we must stop, go find our mate, and attack him, perhaps in a similar way to that in the book. Maybe we just tell him about the scene as we touch him, or maybe we read it to him as he touches us. In any case, we can use the book to enhance our mood, but then we must be sure to share it with our mate. The point is not to simply take care of ourselves (i.e., masturbate) but to include our partner as well, thus improving the passion in our *relationship*.

Members of a book group can also have a lot of fun competing to come up with sexy novels of literary worth or at least books that have some intellectual depth in addition to their romantic value. One of my favorite novelists in this category is Jo Beverley. Beverley's books provide historical accuracy as well as some intelligent plot and dialogue. She is listed along with other romance novelists under "Passion Seekers' Author and Magazine Picks" in the back of this book.

The search for quality X-rated movies has been much more difficult. Tastes and tolerances are so varied that I hesitate to recommend even those titles that are often listed in online surveys I have conducted. Many friends have suggested sticking with more mainstream sexy flicks such as *The Postman Always Rings Twice, Body Heat, Basic Instinct, 9½ Weeks, Wild Orchid, Unfaithful, The Lover,* and *Two Moon Junction.* Movies can be a great Passion Seekers' topic. Once we hear about a flick that might benefit our mood, we should share it with our mate in a "bedroom date night," along with some wine, chocolates, lingerie, etc. I suggest nudity and a great deal of petting during the movie.

I also highly recommend a field trip with friends to the local adult bookstore. My friends and I tried this, and it was great fun. (We even rented a limo and went barhopping afterward.) Some of us were amazed by the variety of products on the market. Just the visit itself was educational. Another way to explore the sex-related products available to us is to invite a representative from an adult store to one of our get-togethers. An at-home showing may be a private and comfortable way to consider the many existing options. With our partner, we can also peruse reputable Web sites (see "Interesting Web Sites" in the back of this book) that sell sex-related products.

A "white-elephant sex toy" gift exchange is another Passion Seekers' party favorite. Everyone brings a new wrapped sex toy to exchange. The fun comes from watching others open the gifts and seeing what each person got. Sometimes an explanation of the item's use is in order. After the party, everyone gets to go home and try the gift out with their mate.

Another support-group activity is to use the Passion Seekers' anonymous survey. This can be found on PassionSeekers.com (under "Passion Poll"). Everyone fills out the survey, and then the answers are read to the group. No one will know who wrote what, and people will hopefully go home with a great idea to try with their mate! It is a lot of fun to hear how everyone answered the questions — often the resulting discussions turn out to be rather stimulating!

Some of the best times I have ever had at a party were spent playing the Passion Seekers' Party Game. Later in the evening at an adults-only party (after the uptight friends have left or after the work gang has gone home), we can pull out this party game.

We will need three prewrapped gifts. (Making the presents misleading in appearance will only add to the fun.) We then act as game host and read off the topic question for the first round (see "Passion Seekers' Party Game — Topic Questions" below). The guests take turns responding. The person with the best answer — the most significant, unique, bizarre, or shocking response — gets to pick a prize. If there is a dispute, the majority decides the winner. After three rounds, when all the prizes have been claimed, the winner of the next round gets to "steal" one of the gifts from a previous winner. This continues with each subsequent round until all the rounds are complete or until a predetermined ending time has been reached. The three players left with the prizes are the final winners.

Passion Seekers' Party Game — Topic Questions

- What is the most unusual place someone you know has had sex?
- What is the most unusual or kinky fetish you have heard or read about?
- What laws should there be about sex and why?
- What is the worst date you ever had and why?
- What is the worst sexual encounter you ever had and why?
- What is the most embarrassing and/or bizarre thing you ever caught a person or persons doing?
- What is the most embarrassing and/or bizarre thing *you* have been caught doing?
- What is the kinkiest thing you have ever heard of a couple doing?
- What is the wildest thing you or someone you know has ever done on vacation?
- What is the kinkiest thing someone you know did on their honeymoon?
- When and what was the earliest sexual encounter you had?

- What is the weirdest tip you have ever heard about sex?
- What is the best advice you have ever heard about sex?
- What is the wildest sexual thing you have ever done in a public place?
- What would you ask a porn star if given the chance?
- What inanimate object has aroused you or someone you know?

This game and all of the Passion Seekers' activities and ideas are for the fun and intelligent Passion Seeker in all of us. We can always use more fun in our marriages and friendships. Any time we share with others, the depth and intimacy of these relationships are deepened.

Discussion possibilities are endless when it comes to sex and passion. However, as these subjects are so private and personal, I have found three main ground rules are required for any passion quest support group discussion or activity:

The Primary Laws of the Passion Seekers' Club

1. *First and foremost we must respect each other's privacy.* There are hazards involved in sharing. I suggest that especially sensitive information be imparted to only the closest of friends. Some revelations are so sensitive that they could severely jeopardize marriages, careers, and reputations. If a member chooses to share such detail, that person's disclosure must stay with the group. Confidentiality is crucial. Our friends must be able to trust us.

2. *We must not hold man-hater meetings or bad-mouth the opposite sex.* Too many times in conversations with women, I have found that discussions about men have turned negative. Once someone starts complaining about "what pigs the guys are," the conversations turn ugly and no one benefits. This sort of discussion may help people blow off a little

steam, but the mood turns negative, and the goal of creating more passion in our lives — specifically with our mate — is defeated. Therefore I advocate having *man-lover* meetings or discussions. This way we can appreciate what he *has* done for us lately and can share positive experiences instead.

3. *We must recognize that all relationships go through peaks and valleys, and if we are in a valley, we need to feed off our friends' peaks.* Each of us experiences low points in our long-term relationship, and the purpose of the support group is to help us through these times and get us on our way toward climbing back up the hill again. And if we *are* experiencing some passion at home, we need to motivate and inspire our friends.

The goal is to always remember the importance of a healthy and active sex life with our mate. The rewards in all aspects of our life will be *huge!*

Our sexual relationship with our mate will greatly benefit from a girls' night out or any form of passion quest support meeting, party, or activity. I have witnessed the effects of such gatherings time and time again. In fact, the results have been so well received by our mates at home that they actually encourage and urge us to take part in any such passion quest events. The point is to have some fun and in the process rediscover the passion and increase the intimacy in our marriages, our friendships, and our lives.

THE PERSISTENT PURSUIT OF PASSION

A support group is vital to our ultimate success in the quest for passion. We can read this book and implement some changes in our sex life or put some effort into heating things up, but after a while we may find it too easy to allow the routine to creep back in and mediocrity to again take hold. To avoid this and reinforce our commitment, we have to make a pact with friends to inspire and support one another in our efforts to keep the passion alive in our relationship.

> The never-ending passion quest is the reward — the pleasure, the intimacy, and the excitement that we are entitled to receive in loving someone until death do us part.

After that first martini meeting with my friends, when we finally spilled the beans to one another about our sex lives (or in some cases the lack thereof), we all experienced a new beginning, or a rebirth, in our long-term relationships. However, it was not too long before a few of the women dropped out and others took their place. Those who never again participated in our Passion Seekers' parties are back to the same old routine and malaise in their relationship. I know this because some of them have told me as much. The rest I have observed with their mates, listening to these women make snide comments about their sex lives and hearing the unhappy comments their mates make to both my husband and me.

I have received e-mails through my Web site from both women and men, complaining that their sex life is boring again and has returned to the routine. When I ask these people if they are doing anything to remedy the boredom and if they have put together a Passion Seekers' support group, they always answer no to both. They make some excuse about how it is their mate's turn to put some effort into lovemaking and then blame their partner for what is not happening in the bedroom. Thus, their quest is not going anywhere.

We must take the lead, get creative, and put some effort into our sex life, but the point is not to do so just once or twice or even for a month but rather to do so *for the life of our relationship.* The pursuit of passion must be persistent, continuous, and never ending. To cease in this endeavor is to suck the passion and eventually the life out of any relationship.

This is not a chore, such as cooking, that we must complete to keep the relationship fed. This is in fact the reward — the pleasure, the intimacy, and the excitement that we are entitled to receive in loving someone until death do us part. If we, or our mate, do not view sex in this way, then we need to try something new — something from this book or from our own creative repertoire. We must also *seek a support group of friends* — friends who will encourage us to seek passion.

We can no longer just sit around and complain about our mate and joke about married sex — or the lack thereof. The divorce rates are too high (see "The Current Estimates for the United States" in chapter 1). Too many people are just plain miserable with the sex in their married existence, and many are having affairs. Without an active and exciting sex life with our mate, we are sacrificing the opportunity to cultivate intimacy, pleasure, and meaningful depth in our marriage.

So *we* must take the initiative — start our own Passion Seekers' support group to put some focus back on our sex life with our mate. The fun and good times this will bring will make us happier and more relaxed, and perhaps make us better parents, workers, and friends. And, of course, the rewards in all aspects of our most important long-term relationship will be huge!

CHAPTER ELEVEN

THE NEVER-ENDING PASSION QUEST

A PASSIONATE LIFETIME WITH OUR MATE

There is a similar thread running through the lives of Nora, Jessie, Carla, Courtney, and Lisa. Each one professed a feeling of boredom and loss of passion in her relationship with her long-term mate. Jessie did not even consciously realize the problem at first, but the loss was there just the same.

For these women, the length of the long-term relationship and the consuming role of parenthood were not the causes of their boredom in the bedroom. Carla had been married only three years, and those with empty nests, such as Nora, were also experiencing problems. These problems were not due to the fact that Courtney and Lisa were housewives without enough to do. In fact, they had arguably the most exhausting and trying of jobs. The problems did not occur because Jessie and Carla were "out there" in the workforce, meeting lots of new and different men.

Rather, Nora, Jessie, Carla, Lisa, and Courtney were discovering that their attitude about sex, their misdirected external quests for answers, and their failure to place any priority on their sex lives at home seriously contributed to the problem. With lessons learned the hard way in some cases, they discovered that a more constructive approach was to improve their attitude, put more effort into their sex life with their long-term mate, and open their heart and mind to what was right there in front of them.

Each of these women took a new look at themselves and their relationship. They discovered how their attitude toward sex with their mate was contributing to, if not causing, a great deal of their discontent. They began to recognize their innate needs and fully utilize their creativity, placing real priority and effort on their most intimate and important relationship.

As I recorded the journeys of these and other women, I found it fascinating to discover that mainstream themes and ideas filtered through even the most extreme scenarios. When I shared these stories with my support group, we were able to glean tidbits of relationship wisdom that made perfect sense for anyone in a long-term relationship. The journeys we take to rediscover the passion are uniquely ours, but the resulting discoveries allow for some universal observations. Below is a summary of what Passion Seekers have learned to apply to any quest for passion:

Passion Seekers' Travel Advice

- If you wait until you have time to travel, the journey will never take place.

- If you ignore the need for a passion quest, the quest may happen without you.
- The travel brochures are misleading. Do your own research.
- Researching a passion quest can be as fun as the trip itself.
- Keep your travel partner's needs in mind and try to accommodate those needs.
- For any quest for passion, pack a positive attitude and an open mind.
- If you place a high priority on your quest for passion, you will reap large rewards.
- Roadblocks and detours are inevitable. Expect them and work around them.
- Continually seek out creative adventures on your road to passion.
- The road less traveled may be exciting but also more dangerous.
- To stray into the land of infidelity will be perilous and possibly fatal for your relationship.
- The more effort you put into the quest, the more you will get out of it.
- Rely on a support group to encourage a continuous quest for passion.
- Always believe that more exciting travels await you and your mate. The best is yet to come.

MOTIVATION TO TRAVEL
AND THE TRAVELER'S FRAME OF MIND

In applying the wisdom we gained from sharing in the journeys of others, we understand that, for most women, sex and intimacy are about what is in our head — how we feel about ourselves and how we choose to see our mate and our relationship. This concept does not have to be complicated. We have control over our own thoughts. We can choose to focus on the "pot of gold" solutions. If we utilize our instinct, our attitude, and our creativity, we will produce renewed desire and satisfaction in the bedroom, and we will ultimately achieve the "feel great" intimacy we crave.

Nevertheless, most of us have experienced difficulty in getting motivated to make any sort of dramatic change. For example, we may want to lose weight. Our partner may also be overweight, yet he continues to eat what he wants instead of what he should be eating. As a result, we find it hard to follow our own diet because we are spending so much time around our chocolate-cake-eating spouse.

The same holds true for our sex life. It is hard to get motivated and take the lead to make a change — even such a fun one — when our mate is still following the same old script. He may not be making much of an attempt to spice things up. He may be slow in responding to our new efforts. He may even reject them at first. However, in time, if we choose to take the lead, we will make a difference. When we stop buying junk food for the house, he will find it harder to eat it. When we start exercising and losing weight, he will eventually take notice. Sex is no different. When we stop the routine and start implementing a new frame of mind, things will start to change. The journey will begin anew.

As we saw in the real-life examples in this book, getting motivated to take a quest for passion in our long-term relationship requires adjusting our attitude to a traveler's frame of mind:

How to Ensure You Do Not Go Anywhere	How to Ensure Exciting Journeys to Passionville
Smile as you walk down the aisle, knowing you just gave your last blow job.	Smile as you walk down the aisle, thinking of all the sexual adventures that await you.
Take off all your makeup and dress comfortably before he gets home.	Freshen up your face before he gets home and wear something nice.
Deny your innate travel spirit.	Listen to your innate desires to take a journey seeking passion.
Ignore your mate.	Date your mate.
Never plan any sexual adventures.	Take the lead and act as a travel guide to passion.
Overlook how your past travels haunt you (chapters 6 and 7).	Rediscover or redirect the passion within.
Stay in familiar territory.	Head down a new and different path.
Assume you know all there is to know about your travel partner.	Continually get reacquainted with your travel partner. Try the Passion Seekers' research ideas in chapter 9.
Take excess baggage on your journey (see chapter 2).	Check the excess baggage and, if you must, claim it after you have had sex.
Take a journey later when the kids are grown or when you have more time.	Take a journey while you still have a travel partner.
Go to the same place every time.	Seek out someplace new.
Stay on the bus and miss all the sights.	Get off the bus and explore the possibilities!

If a change is ever going to happen, someone has to adjust his or her attitude and take the lead — and how empowering it is to be the instigator! Our actions will inspire our mate. Change may not be easy at first, but the payoff will come. He will take notice and likely follow suit. Things will get more interesting — we have the power to make it so!

DETOURS, DEAD ENDS, AND THE END OF THE ROAD

Unfortunately, there is always the possibility that our actions will go unnoticed. Or worse, he may even insult our efforts, laugh at them, or ignore them. There is also the possibility that what we do will never make a difference. Seeking to improve passion is not going to solve bigger problems. There are negative relationships that require much more than improving sexual intimacy. Passion is only a piece of the puzzle, and we need the complete frame to hold it all together.

At least in regard to rekindling the passion, as with the weight-loss example, we will be able to hold our head high and be proud of the efforts we have made as Passion Seekers. We can be sure that we did not stick our head in the sand. We did what we could. We took action. We are better people for it, and if our relationship has a loving and trusting foundation (and no additional big issues to deal with), our life with our mate will ultimately be much better for it.

In twenty, thirty, or forty years from now, when we look back over our time with our mate, how will we feel? Will we be full of regret? Will we wonder how our life might have been different? Will we think about what we should have done or what we could have done? Will all the "would've, should've, could'ves" haunt us? Or will we know we gave it our best?

I know someone whose husband passed away. She told me that the worst place to be in old age is not one of loneliness but of regret. In their marriage, she was in a constant state of conflict with her mate — control issues controlled them. As time passed, they put less and less effort into having fun alone together. They never took the time to really listen and give to each other in the bedroom and out of it. Now it was too late, and her husband died never knowing that she regretted all the lost moments of pleasure and intimacy.

With a *"stagnant* quo" in place, pushing the fast-forward button and seeing the end result may not be a pretty sight. We may at some point realize that we missed out and that we did not do the best we could have done. Nobody wants to be in that place. We want to be proud of our efforts and not have to wonder, *If only we had . . .* or *If only we had not . . .*

If we are lucky — and if we really work at it — the passion quest will be never ending, but that does not mean there will never be delays and detours. We may need to seek professional help to struggle against these issues and brilliantly deal with them, but the problems may nevertheless end up defeating our relationship. There are those unfortunate events and serious issues that may occur, and if the problems are truly insurmountable, sometimes the journey ends for good. Sometimes things do not work out the way we planned and we have to face the shortcomings of reality.

The journey may come to an early end with our mate despite all of our efforts — despite placing a high priority on passion. Sometimes all the creativity and all the energy we put into it are never going to be enough. Even with the best-planned adventure, some just never reach the destinations of choice, and some never even get off the ground at all. The trip turns into a nightmare.

If we face the insurmountable and end up on a journey by ourselves, we must recognize that although the passion quest (among other things) failed, we can learn through this failure how to plan a better route next time. We may pack differently. We might understand how to avoid the pitfalls. We can now start out another day, with more chances to travel and other passion quests to embark on. There is *always* another route to take — another train coming, another flight out, another adventure waiting for us.

It is always sad to have to end a journey and wonder if and when we will have the time or energy to begin a new one. But through this sadness and uncertainty will come that fresh beginning — the passion of a new, exciting relationship that will benefit from the wisdom of an experienced traveler.

We now know that delays and detours will always occur, no matter how much effort we put into planning our trip. The experienced traveler understands that these hassles are always going to be there. For a passion quest to stay on course, we must continually pay attention to where we are heading and map out the best way to get there. We must accept the delays and detours with grace and dignity — and continue on our way.

THE NEVER-ENDING PASSION QUEST

Without a journey seeking passion in our life, our relationship may exist just fine — but it exists without going anywhere. Our long-term relationship becomes stagnant and routine. New destinations and ongoing journeys are the only ways to expand the horizon and continually achieve fun, intimacy, pleasure, and peace. We can choose to invest in all the latest travel gear or just take that first little step toward seeking passion — either way, the trip is worth taking.

> There are a lot of problems that can break up a marriage, but if effort is put into passionately making love, this can go a long way toward easing the other issues.

Enjoying ourselves in a long-term relationship necessitates that we continually seek passion with our mate. We cannot — even during the busiest stages of our life — put off the journey or expect that it will happen on its own. We must not sit back and hope someone else carries us along or plans the next leg of the trip for us. We especially cannot avoid the journey altogether, thinking there will always be time to travel later. We will miss out on too much. The passion will fizzle out, and the quest will likely become permanently grounded.

There is no better time to travel than right now. The fares will never be lower. Life is too short to hold off on the pleasure, fun, and intimacy that come from seeking passion with our long-term mate. We cannot wait until we have more time and energy — that day may never come. Rather, the moment for a passion quest with our mate is now, *today*. There is no better time to fly.

Many years from now, will we reminisce about our relationship and smile, remembering all the intimate moments of pleasure and joy we shared? Or will we look back and regret a passionless marriage? Worse yet, will we have lost that mate to divorce, and wonder *If only . . .* or *Should we have . . . ?* The passion in our long-term relationship is a burning fire. At first, the flame is bright and strong, but eventually we must tend to it, throw another log on it, and continually ensure that the fire does not go out.

I hope our long-term relationship will be one in which our gifts will be utilized to the fullest — in which the thought that "something's missing" does not haunt us once the newness wears off; in which creative effort, intellectual stimulation, and emotional commitment continually fuel and renew the passion; and in which, above all, we get a feeling of "I am home," a warm comfort that comes from being truly accepted regardless of imperfections, idiosyncrasies, and insecurities.

May my hope be our reality.

GLOSSARY

THE PASSION SEEKERS' GUIDE TO THE LINGO

This glossary will help us keep up with the language every sexually well-informed person should know. It is obviously not meant to be exhaustive; I am not presenting a lexicon of words or topics on sexuality. Rather, this glossary is a fun girlfriends' guide to identifying and defining words and phrases commonly used to describe modern-day sexual escapades, along with suggestions and pointers.

I discovered these words and phrases — mostly slang — during my research into the sex lives of wives. Incorporated in the definitions are summaries of both conventional usages found in standard dictionaries and common usages from popular Internet sites. Also defined are a few words and phrases coined by the Passion Seekers themselves.

Aphrodisiac: Something that arouses, increases, or intensifies sexual desire. Examples include oysters (to eat), chocolate (also to eat, preferably off each other), Coppertone suntan oil (for the aroma and to use with a massage), lilacs (for their fragrance), and, of course, attendance at a Passion Seekers' party.

BDSM: Bondage, discipline, sadism, masochism (see also each term, separately defined in this glossary). "BDSM" commonly refers to the erotic *and* consensual exchange of power between a sadist, or dominant, and masochist, or submissive, to obtain sexual pleasure and satisfaction, usually through the use of bondage and discipline. For a fairly encyclopedic explanation of BDSM, go to en.wikipedia.org/wiki/BDSM.

Bedroom attire: No, sweats and pajamas do not count as bedroom attire. Rather, the term refers to sexy clothing that is appropriate to wear only in private — whatever makes *us* feel sexy.

Bi-curious: An individual who has no experience with same-sex encounters but who is interested in exploring them.

Big "O": An orgasm or the act of reaching sexual climax.

Bi-playful: An individual who has no problem with same-sex touching or mild interaction but who has no real attraction to the same sex; often used to refer to two women interacting in a sexy manner for the purpose of arousing a man (or men).

Bisexual: An individual who is interested and aroused sexually by both males and females but typically has a stronger preference for one or the other.

Bondage: Mainstream bondage involves being tied up or restrained for pleasure, using such items as scarves, neckties, housecoat belts, and furry handcuffs. The recipient, or the person tied up, is sexually teased, etc., while the partner gets to have his or her way with the restrained person. In BDSM (see term in this glossary) practices, the submissive person is physically restricted from movement through the use of such materials as plastic wrap, duct tape, or rope.

Brazilian style: A Brazilian bikini wax involves having all the hair in the genital area removed. "Brazilian style" is the term Passion Seekers use to refer to the practice of offering sex to one's mate with a fully shaved or fully waxed bikini area.

Cat-o'-nine-tails: This is a type of whip used in erotic play and flagellation (see term in this glossary). It is often referred to as simply a "cat" — a whip with multiple tails that are usually braided. Although commonly used in hard-core BDSM (see term in this glossary) play, adult novelty stores carry a variety of choices, including soft-touch whips for more mainstream use.

Cheating: (Also infidelity, adultery, "going out on one's spouse," unfaithfulness, double-crossing, getting involved in extra-curricular activities or an illicit affair, moonlighting, sneaking around, two-timing, being unchaste.) Often defined as the immoral behavior of having emotional and/or physical involvement with someone who is not one's spouse and then lying to one's spouse about it.

Come home to eat: Monogamous in all physical ways. Note the expression "It does not matter where we get our appetite as long as we come home to eat," meaning arousal due to outside sources does not matter as long as we relieve such arousal only with our mate at home.

Consensual power exchange: The preferred characterization of common uses of BDSM (see term in this glossary) play.

Cowgirl sex: (Also reverse missionary style, Amazon, and "riding your man.") Slang for having the woman on top during sexual intercourse. Such a sexual position is considered to enhance genital stimulation for women.

Creative expeditions: Used by Passion Seekers to refer to the vast and endless passion quest possibilities we are able to create in our own bedroom if we break out of our routine and train our mind to think of sex as a form of art in which our creativity may blossom and be released (see chapter 4).

Cultural arts: Term found on the Internet and in personal ads that refers to an individual's sexual-technique preferences. Users commonly indicate such preferences through listing the names of the nationalities that are loosely (and stereotypically) associated with different tendencies, including English (to refer to spanking), French (to refer to oral), German (to refer to discipline), Greek (to refer to anal), and Swedish (to refer to manual).

Cunnilingus: (Also muff diving, pussy eating, carpet munching, dining at the Y, eating her out, a box lunch, beaver munching, clit licking, sugar time [between just women], cunt licking, feasting on tuna, and going south.) Term for "going down on" a woman, meaning to suck on her genitals.

Cybersex: (Also cybering and virtual sex.) When two or more people connected through the Internet — often through chat rooms and instant messaging — exchange a series of sexually explicit messages describing themselves and various sexual acts. Cybersex is similar to "phone sex" but is even more anonymous and impersonal (except, of course, when video cameras are used). When performed without the knowledge of one's spouse, cybersex is considered by some to be the same as "cheating."

Dirty story: As in "Tell me a dirty story" — a great way to initiate a sexual encounter with one's mate. The dirty story can be any sexually explicit tale.

Discipline: Used in BDSM (see term in this glossary) practice to refer to the action used when the dominant person physically corrects or punishes the submissive partner for his or her failure to behave. In more mainstream erotic role-playing, discipline is used in a lighthearted manner in the acting out of a dominant-submissive fantasy such as that of a "student" being reprimanded by the "teacher."

Doggie style: Although well-known slang for the sexual position of a woman on all fours with the man entering her from behind, the term is included here because there are some girlfriends unfamiliar with this position (and missing out on a lot of fun).

Earn our wings: Having sex on an airplane will "earn us our wings." (See "mile-high club" in this glossary.)

English style: A type of "cultural art" (see term in this glossary). If people say they like or want sex "English style," they are usually referring to spanking or being spanked, or some other form of erotic discipline play as part of lovemaking.

Erotica: As opposed to commercial pornography, "erotica" includes any media with sexual content — usually stories, photos, and films — that attempt or attain a higher quality of artistic depth.

Exhibitionist: In a sexual context, the term commonly refers to an individual or couple who likes to be watched while having sex. It may also be used to describe someone who shows off to attract sexual attention. (Note: This is different from the actual psychiatric disorder involving a compulsion to show one's genitals in public.)

Experimentation: Passion Seekers welcome and encourage sexual experimentation for the health and welfare of our most important long-term relationship, whether this means making love in the shower, using props, or taking a vacation alone together. Experimentation is the key to any quest for passion.

Eye candy: Anyone attractive or pleasing to look at, as in "a treat for the eyes."

Fantasy location sex: Creating a faraway place in our bedroom at home, either through storytelling or the use of props. For example, we can have "sex on the beach" by sipping fruity drinks (try Passion Seekers' Punch [see term in this glossary]); playing tropical music, an ocean-sounds CD, or an ocean-scenes DVD; lighting tropical-scented candles; starting out in our swimwear and spreading coconut oil on each other, etc.

Fellatio: (Also blow job, giving head, "going down on," cock sucking, shines [UK], hummer, slobber on the bobber, and French style [see term in this glossary].) Term for sucking on his genitals.

Flagellation: (Also English style [see term in this glossary].) The act of spanking, whipping, or paddling in an erotic context, sometimes softly (repeatedly) and sometimes forcefully. Used commonly in BDSM (see term in this glossary) impact play on the submissive person.

Foreplay: Stimulating interaction before intercourse. Yes, foreplay *can* be reintroduced into a long-term relationship. We can try setting the example by tying up our mate and teasing him to the point of exasperation or just spending some time making out while our clothing is still on.

French style: A type of "cultural art" (see term in this glossary). If people say they like or want sex "French style," they are usually referring to oral sex (see "cunnilingus" and "fellatio" in this glossary).

German style: A type of "cultural art" (see term in this glossary). If people say they like or want sex "German style," they are usually referring to using discipline or BDSM (see term in this glossary).

Greek style: A type of "cultural art" (see term in this glossary). If people say they like or want sex "Greek style," they usually mean they enjoy anal sex.

G-spot: Named after German gynecologist Ernst Grafenberg, the G-spot is not imaginary but is an actual part of the female genitals located behind the pubic bone in the tissue surrounding the urethra. When stimulated directly, it is believed to create a more intense orgasm. The fun is in searching for it.

Hand play: This term includes not just the act of masturbating but also caressing, inserting, massaging, pinching, restraining, rubbing, scratching, spanking, squeezing, tickling, or anything else we can use our hands for while making love.

Imaginary playmates: Used by Passion Seekers to refer to a virtual ménage à trois. The sensuous use of voice and imagination takes our mate into the fantasy of having another person in the bedroom. We tell a story, softly and sensually describing to our mate an imaginary visitor in our bedroom and what this person is doing, at the same time actually doing it (making sure our approach is different from our routine). Or we can tell our mate what he is doing to this visitor as he does it to us. (This is a great way to subtly let him know what we want in the bedroom.)

Infidelity: Commonly used to refer to unfaithfulness or the failure to fulfill the physical or emotional sexual commitment of a monogamous relationship. Different people have different ideas on what sort of behavior constitutes infidelity: some define the term as sexual intercourse or any sexual contact with anyone other than one's mate, and some add cybersex and even flirting to their interpretation. It might be helpful to have a clear understanding with our mate regarding what constitutes infidelity in our relationship. (See "cheating" in this glossary.)

Kama Sutra: The Kama Sutra is an ancient Indian guide (believed to have been written sometime between the first and sixth centuries) to enjoying sexual relations on a deeper level. It includes erotic technique, sixty-four sex positions, kissing, foreplay, oral sex, orgasm, and more. There are a number of Web sites with animation of the positions from the Kama Sutra.

Key party: Used in the world of swinging (see term in this glossary) during the 1960s and 1970s to refer to a party in which the male guests would put their car keys in a bowl, and then the women would each select a set to see which vehicle owner she would go home with. Today, the term is infrequently used, and usually only in jest.

Kinky sex play: Anything commonly considered outside mainstream sexual practices. The term usually refers to highly unconventional sexual acts.

Lifestyle: The modern term used to describe a heterosexual couple's repeated practice of swinging (see term in this glossary), which typically means that two couples exchange partners for the purpose of sexual interaction.

Lifestylers: Couples who live the "lifestyle" (see term in this glossary).

Location sex: Sex anywhere but in our usual bed in our home. Suggested locations to have sex include on the floor, in the shower, on a chair, in the backyard in the middle of the night, on the beach, in the bathroom at a party, in the car while "parking" with our mate, at a hotel, in the woods, on the hood of our car, on a boat, on the golf course late at night, in the hot tub or Jacuzzi, behind locked doors at the office, under the desk, up against a wall, on a raft, in the ocean, on a plane, in the janitor's closet, under the bleachers, on the ski lift, on the mountain, etc.

Love bite: Another term for a hickey — a temporary mark on the skin resulting from strong kissing and sucking in one place, usually on the neck.

Masochist/Masochism: A masochist is someone who receives sexual pleasure or gratification from being emotionally and/or physically abused. When referring to an actual *need* for pain, masochism may be considered a psychological disorder.

Mile-high club: We become members of the "mile-high club" by having sexual relations on an airplane and therefore "earning our wings" (see term in this glossary). There is actually an association that offers flights in which private couches or beds are included — go to milehighclub.com.

MILF: An acronym for Mother I'd Like to F—k. To be called a MILF is actually a compliment, especially when our mate says it in reference to us.

Missionary position: We all know this common sexual position, but the key is to try as many variations on it as we can conjure up, including placing pillows under our rear, placing our legs up on his shoulders, or just reaching and stroking unusual places with our hands while in this position.

Monogamous: A sexual relationship with only one partner.

Mouth play: Involves kissing and sucking our partner's various body parts but also includes love biting, blowing, licking, flicking with the tongue, nibbling, and swirling motions with the tongue, using a wide range of pressure and intensity.

Nude beach: As opposed to a "prude beach," any beach where clothing is legally optional or is not allowed at all. There are nude beaches at a number of adults-only resorts, especially in the Caribbean and Mediterranean regions. According to travelchannel.com (2005), some of the world's best nude beaches are Montalivet, France; Ocho Rios, Jamaica; Wreck Beach, British Columbia; Samurai Beach, Australia; Hedonism II, Jamaica; Praia do Pinho, Brazil; Red Beach, Greece; Haulover Beach, Florida; Red, White, and Blue Beach, California; and Little Beach, Hawaii.

Obligatory leg spread: When a woman has sex with her mate even when she does not want to because she feels it is her duty as a spouse.

Open relationship/marriage: A nonmonogamous long-term relationship; a couple who remains in a long-term relationship but agrees to allow each other to have independent sexual contact and even sexual relationships with third parties.

Passion: Used in this book to mean strong sexual desire, enthusiasm, and excitement.

Passion quest or journey: Passion Seekers define this term as an effort to actively seek out and create passionate and intimate sexual encounters with one's mate in a long-term relationship.

Passion quest support group: The group of friends with whom we can actually open up, share, and feel supported by in our effort to rediscover the passion in our marriage and long-term relationship. My passion quest support group eventually evolved into the Passion Seekers' Club, which anyone may become a part of by visiting PassionSeekers.com.

Passion Seekers and the Passion Seekers' Club: Any group of people who wish to get together periodically to support one another in the effort to keep their long-term relationship and sex life healthy and thriving. Members exchange ideas and stories, and participate in games and partylike get-togethers that remind them of the benefits — to themselves, their relationship, and their family — of continually seeking passion in their long-term relationship. Remember the Passion Seekers' Motto: Seeking the passion in our relationship will send us on the road to a happier, healthier, and more relaxed self. We must enjoy ourselves while we still can and our relationship while we still have it!

Passion Seekers' Punch: Equal parts quality vodka and purple grape juice (not grape drink or soda) with ½ part of Cointreau and a splash of sweet and sour. Shake with ice to chill and serve in a martini glass, or blend for a slushy drink and garnish with an orange slice.

Passionville: Used by Passion Seekers to refer to the choice destination of any passion quest — that figurative place (or literal state) of sexual excitement, great sex, and dynamic intimacy.

Penis: (Also baby maker, cock, dick, dong, dork, fire hose, hose, johnson, joystick, knob, manhood, member, one-eyed monster, one-eyed snake, package, pecker, peepee, peter, phallus, prick, rod, sausage, schlong, schmuck, todger, tool, trouser snake, wang, weenie, wiener, and willy.) The large number of slang terms for the penis (primarily used by men) might give us a clue as to the importance men place on their genitals and the time put in to thinking about (and with) them. A fun icebreaker at our next Passion Seekers' party would be to have our guests come up with as many slang terms for "penis" as possible. (We can get creative with the prize for the person with the highest number. For example, a penis-shaped thermos from our local adult store or a dildo might be appropriate.)

Perform: Sometimes used in a negative manner, as in "I have to 'perform' for [put out for or have sex with] my mate tonight." However, a Passion Seeker might say, "I cannot wait to perform for my mate tonight. I have a fabulous production planned. . . ."

Perilous journey: A Passion Seekers' term meaning risking one's relationship with an illicit affair (see "cheating" in this glossary). Also refers to the act of dancing on the edge of infidelity and the risks involved in doing so.

Pet penis philosophy/approach: Passion Seekers' lingo for the technique of treating our mate's genitals as well as we do our dog or cat — with affection, praise, and attention throughout the day, resulting in complete devotion to us, its owner.

Phone sex: This practice is often forgotten in long-term relationships. Passion Seekers recommend reviving the well-known technique of talking sexy over the phone with our mate when we cannot be with him. This is a great tool for sharing sexual fantasies.

Porno: Short for "pornographic," or any sexually explicit media intended to cause sexual arousal.

Promiscuous: Commonly means having numerous casual sexual relationships but is sometimes used to describe a couple who agrees to an "open relationship" or "swinging" (see terms in this glossary).

Prude beach: Any beach that does not allow nudity.

Quickie: Having sexual intercourse quickly, as in "Please join me for a quickie." Sometimes this is a good thing.

Role-playing: The act of playing a role during sex to create a fantasy or a mood. We should think of it as make-believe play for adults. For role-playing suggestions, see "Passion Seekers' Role-Playing Ideas" in chapter 4.

Rough sex: Consensual wild and nasty sex with possible biting, forceful tossing around, spanking, scratching, etc. As opposed to gentle and romantic, rough sex appears violent. It is common in BDSM (see term in this glossary) practices and may verge on brutal or possibly painful interactions.

Sadist/Sadism: A sexual sadist literally gains sexual arousal and satisfaction from being mentally and/or physically abusive to his or her partner. When referring to an actual *need* to do this, sadism may be considered a psychological disorder.

Safeword: A word or phrase agreed upon in advance as a safety precaution to stop the action, role-play, bondage, or discipline in BDSM (see term in this glossary) play, typically used by the submissive participant when they have reached their limit.

Serial monogamist: Any person who has a continual series of monogamous relationships, one after another. Typically a "serial monogamist" is a person who has a pattern of ending a relationship when the going gets rough or the passion wanes, instead of putting the effort into making things work long-term.

Sex slave: A fun gift to give our mate is to offer ourselves as a "sex slave" for a set period of time, doing whatever our mate tells us to do. Receiving such a gift is great fun as well.

Sexual fetish: A Freudian concept but usually used today to refer to an object or a body part that a person has extraordinary attachment to or affection for. Common sexual fetishes include feet, breasts, lingerie, spandex, leather, rubber, fur, body piercing, and shoes.

Skin magazine: Any magazine that contains nude photos or pornographic images.

Spicy: If a couple has a "spicy" relationship, they are probably Passion Seekers. "Keeping it spicy" means creatively and actively working on seeking passion — keeping things lively — in our long-term relationship.

Stepford wife: From the novel by Ira Levin, meaning a spouse perfectly engineered to meet her husband's every need and desire. Used by Passion Seekers in a derogatory manner to refer to someone who just puts out for her mate out of a sense of duty, does not ask for what she wants, and fails to take any lead in creating a passionate relationship *and* a passionate self — or just does so to please her mate (as opposed to recognizing her own needs as well).

Sublimation: Used by Passion Seekers to refer to either the positive act of channeling or redirecting undesirable strong sexual impulses into more acceptable activities (as in Carla's case) or the detrimental displacement of our passionate needs and desires into everything *but* our long-term sexual relationship.

Swedish style: A type of "cultural art" (see term in this glossary). If people say they like or want sex "Swedish style," they are usually referring to manual sex, which is the use of hand play (see term in this glossary) on someone's genitals to achieve orgasm.

Swinging: (Also swapping.) Typically means that two couples exchange partners for sexual interaction with the other's mate. Many swingers indicate that true swinging requires that one fully share the encounter with one's spouse in the same room. Also may be loosely used to refer to a couple who invites *any* outsider(s) into their bed.

Taboo: The sexually taboo is any prohibited and forbidden sexual act. What is taboo to one person, couple, or group may not be to another.

Three-way: A ménage à trois (French for "household of three") — any sexual act involving three people.

Toys: Refers to any sexual prop or apparatus used to enhance a sexual encounter. Common store-bought toys include vibrators, dildos, cock rings, butt plugs or beads, and warming lotions. A great Web site for toys is goodvibes.com (or call 1-800-BUY-VIBE). Homemade toys might include feather dusters, silk scarves, whipped cream, Pam spray, vegetable oil, ice, etc.

Vacation-anticipation sex: Occurs when eagerly preparing for and looking forward to an upcoming vacation alone with our mate increases the excitement in our sexual encounters together.

Vacation sex: Literally means the great and passionate sex we have when we are on vacation. Participants from survey after survey on my Web site agree that sex on vacation is better, more exciting, and more satisfying. When we are on vacation we are more relaxed, have more time and energy, and have our focus on the moment.

Vanilla sex: Conventional, mainstream sex, usually experienced in the missionary position, as opposed to, for example, sex in unusual positions or locations, fetish play, the use of props, swinging, threesomes, BDSM play, or any other such "wild explorations" (see term in this glossary).

Visual stimulation: Anything that we can see that will sexually stimulate us or our mate. In many cases, men are extremely "visually stimulated," and therefore anything we can do to make ourselves look sexually appealing may inspire passion in our mate, as might skin magazines and porno movies (see terms in this glossary).

Voyeur: Term for someone who likes to watch others while they are having sex.

White-bread: Derisive slang used to describe white mainstream American culture. Typically it is believed that someone who is "white-bread" is into only "vanilla sex" (see term in this glossary), but this is not necessarily the case. We never really know what goes on behind closed doors.

Wild explorations: Used in this book to refer to sexual practices that are typically and traditionally considered outside the mainstream or are otherwise unconventional.

THE PASSION SEEKERS' GUIDE TO SEXY ENTERTAINMENT

PASSION SEEKERS' AUTHOR AND MAGAZINE PICKS

Austen, Jane

Beverley, Jo (intelligent historical romance novels — wonderfully romantic and sensual, especially the Medieval, Company of Rogues, and Malloren series; jobev.com)

Brontë, Anne, Charlotte, and Emily (classic and romantic)

Friday, Nancy (particularly *Men in Love.* Dell Publishing, 1980; everything you have ever wanted to know about what men fantasize about)

Glyn, Elinor (early-twentieth-century writer)

Penthouse Forum (short sex stories)

Pilcher, Rosamunde (very romantic and very tame)

Playboy Advisor column

Putney, Mary Jo (great romance novels)

Rice, Anne (particularly *Exit to Eden.* Dell Publishing, 1985; sexy romance with glamorized S and M)

Samuel, Barbara, aka Ruth Wind (great romance novels)
Seton, Anya (historical romance novels)
Sparks, Nicholas (bestselling love stories)
(See the resources section for more ideas.)

PASSION SEEKERS' MUSICIAN PICKS

Bach
Barry, John (particularly *Moviola*)
Enigma
Enya (particularly *Watermark*)
Gaye, Marvin
Getz, Stan
Grobin, Josh
Jobim
Jones, Norah (particularly *Come Away with Me*)
Kenny G
Prince (particularly *Purple Rain*)
Ravel (particularly *The Ultimate Bolero*)
Robinson, Smokey
Stewart, Rod
Stone, Josh
Vandross, Luther
White, Barry
Yanni

PASSION SEEKERS' MOVIE PICKS

VERY SEXY (NONPORN)
Basic Instinct, 1992
Blown Away, 1992
Body Heat, 1981
Bound, 1996
Delta of Venus, 1995
The Lover, 1992
9½ Weeks, 1986
Summer Lovers, 1982
Thief of Hearts, 1984
Toute Une Vie (And Now My Love), 1974
Two Moon Junction, 1988
Wild Orchid, 1990

MISCELLANEOUS
ROMANTIC/PASSIONATE
An Affair to Remember, 1957
Casablanca, 1942
Doctor Zhivago, 1965
Ghost, 1990
Gone With the Wind, 1939
The Graduate, 1967
Love Story, 1970
An Officer and a Gentleman, 1982
The Piano, 1993
The Postman Always Rings Twice, 1946

MISCELLANEOUS ROMANTIC/
PASSIONATE (CONT.)
Pretty Woman, 1990
Roman Holiday, 1953
Romeo and Juliet, 1968

Shakespeare in Love, 1998
Unfaithful, 2002
The Way We Were, 1973
West Side Story, 1961
Wuthering Heights, 1939

INTERESTING WEB SITES

adultsonlytravel.com (great vacation ideas)

allsexreviews.com (reviews of sex products and movies)

ameanet.org (Web site of the World Museum of Erotic Art based in Amsterdam; e-mail postcards one can send to one's mate and links to the erotic art world)

clubmed.com (all-inclusive vacation resorts)

customeroticasource.com (people state their preferences and have erotic stories created for them)

fatalemedia.com (Fanny Fatale's line on learning how to female ejaculate)

forthegirls.com (e-zine and erotica for women)

goodvibes.com (great site for sex toys)

ladylynx.com (offers links to adult sites and erotica especially for women)

milehighclub.com (fly and have sex at the same time)

passionparties.com (host a party to see and buy sex toys and related products)

PassionSeekers.com (seek the passion — join our online support group and chat room, and receive marriage-enriching and passion-enhancing ideas and tips!)

superclubs.com (great all-inclusive, adults-only resorts)

tantra.com (Web site containing the text of the Kama Sutra, as well as explanations of positions and accompanying pictures)

RESOURCES

BOOKS, REPORTS, AND STUDIES

Allen, Ed, and Dana Allen. *Together Sex.* Momentpoint Media, 2001. (Complete guide to the "lifestyle.")

Arp, David, and Claudia Arp. *10 Great Dates to Energize Your Marriage.* Zondervan Publishing, 1997.

Atwood, Joan D., and Limor Schwartz. "Cybersex: The New Affair Treatment Considerations." *Journal of Couple and Relationship Therapy,* 1, no. 3 (2002).

Barash, David P., and Judith Eve Lipton. *The Myth of Monogamy.* W. H. Freeman, 2001. (Scientific and technical look at human mating.)

Bramlett, Matthew, and William Mosher. "First Marriage Dissolution, Divorce, and Remarriage: United States." Advance data from vital and health statistics, no. 323. Hyattsville, Maryland: National

Center for Health Statistics, 2001. (See also cdc.gov/od/oc/media/pressrel/r010524.htm)

Cattrall, Kim. *Sexual Intelligence.* Bulfinch Press, 2005. (Explores sexual desire. Beautifully illustrated.)

"Changes in Women's Labor Force Participation in the 20th Century." U.S. Bureau of Labor Statistics, February 16, 2000. (See also bls.gov/opub/ted/2000/feb/wk3/art03.htm)

Cohen, Angela, and Sarah Gardner Fox. *The Wise Woman's Guide to Erotic Videos: 300 Sexy Videos for Every Woman — and Her Lover.* Broadway, 1997.

Easton, Dossie, and Catherine A. Liszt. *The Ethical Slut.* Greenery Press, 1997. (A look at open relationships and free love.)

Hendricks, Gay, and Kathlyn Hendricks. *Lasting Love: The Five Secrets of Growing a Vital, Conscious Relationship.* Rodale, 2004. Also *Spirit-Centered Relationships.* Hay House, 2006.

Janus, Samuel S., and Cynthia L. Janus. *The Janus Report on Sexual Behavior: The First Broadscale Scientific National Survey Since Kinsey.* Reprint. Wiley, 1994.

Kelsey, Dick. "Survey: Variety of Reasons for Cybersex." *Newsbytes,* 2001. Reporting on the 2000 Online Cybersex Survey by MSNBC.com and Dr. Alvin Cooper, director of the San Jose Marital Services and Sexuality Center in California. (See also usatoday.com/tech/nb/nb1.htm)

Kreider, Rose M., and Jason M. Fields. "Number, Timing, and Duration of Marriages and Divorces: 1996." U.S. Census Bureau Current Population Reports (February 2002): 18.

Love, Patricia, and Jo Robinson. *Hot Monogamy.* Plume, 1994. (Therapist's approach, with tests and exercises to fulfilling emotional as well as sexual needs.)

McCarthy, Barry, and Emily McCarthy. *Rekindling Desire: A Step-by-Step Program to Help Low-Sex and No-Sex Marriages.* Taylor & Francis, 2003.

McGraw, Phillip C. *Relationship Rescue: A Seven-Step Strategy for Reconnecting with Your Partner.* Hyperion, 2000.

Munson, Martha, and Paul Sutton. "Births, Marriages, Divorces, and Deaths: Provisional Data for 2003." National vital statistics reports 52, no. 22. Hyattsville, Maryland: National Center for Health Statistics, 2004. (See also cdc.gov/nchs/fastats/divorce.htm)

Page, Susan. The 8 Essential Traits of Couples Who Thrive. Little, Brown and Company, 1994. (Very useful guide.)

————. How One of You Can Bring the Two of You Together. Broadway Books, 1997. (Excellent strategies and encouragement to make a positive impact on one's relationship.)

————. Why Talking Is Not Enough: 8 Loving Actions That Will Transform Your Marriage. Jossey-Bass, 2006.

Réage, Pauline. Story of O. Ballantine Books, 1965. (S and M.)

Sacher-Masoch, Leopold. Venus in Furs. Penguin Classic, 2000. (S and M.)

Schnarch, David. Passionate Marriage. Henry Holt and Company, 1997. (Marriage therapy.)

Smith, Tom W. "American Sexual Behavior: Trends, Socio-Demographic Differences, and Risk Behavior." National Opinion Research Center, University of Chicago. General Social Survey Topical Report, no. 25 (Updated April 2003).

Stuart, Mary. "Infidelity." Divorcetransitions.com/articles/infidelity.htm, July 2000. (Web site of Pen Central Press, publisher of The Divorce Recovery Journal by Linda C. Senn and Mary Stuart, 1999; and Your Pocket Divorce Guide by Linda C. Senn, 1999.)

Taormino, Tristan. Down and Dirty Sex Secrets: The New and Naughty Guide to Being Great in Bed. Regan Books, 2003.

Vaughan, Peggy. The Monogamy Myth: A Personal Handbook for Recovering from Affairs. 3rd ed. Newmarket Press, 2003. (See also dearpeggy.com)

West, David, and Louis James. Adults Only Travel: The Ultimate Guide to Romantic and Erotic Destinations. 2nd ed. Diamond Publishing, 2003. (Excellent source for sexy places to visit with our mate.)

Wiseman, Jay. SM 101: A Realistic Introduction. Greenery Press, 1996. (A complete and shocking instructional manual for the safe practice of sadomasochism.)

SPECIAL RESOURCES

AASECT (American Association of Sex Educators, Counselors, and
Therapists), Web site: aasect.org
National AIDS Hotline: 1-800-342-AIDS, Web site: thebody.com
National STD Hotline: 1-800-227-8922, Web site: ashastd.org
Sexaholics Anonymous, Web site: sa.org
Sex and Love Addicts Anonymous, Web site: slaafws.org
Society for the Scientific Study of Sexuality, Web site: sexscience.org

INDEX

PASSION SEEKERS' COUPONS TO GIVE TO HIM

PASSION SEEKERS' COUPON ♥

This coupon entitles you to one *romantic and passionate date* with your mate, entirely planned and orchestrated by yours truly.

_____ Advance notice required.

PASSION SEEKERS' COUPON ♥

This coupon entitles you to a *fast and frantic f—k* session with yours truly — the tramp.

_____ Advance notice required.

PASSION SEEKERS' COUPON ♥

This coupon entitles you to a *bedroom story* narrated by yours truly.

No advance notice required.

PASSION SEEKERS' COUPON ♥

This coupon entitles you to ___ minutes of *oral sex.*

No advance notice required.

PASSION SEEKERS' COUPON ♥

This coupon entitles you to a *quickie.*

No advance notice required.

PASSION SEEKERS' COUPON ♥

Master, this coupon entitles you to *one half hour of slavery* by yours truly.

No advance notice required.

PASSION SEEKERS' COUPON ♥

Master, this coupon entitles you to *one hour of slavery* by yours truly.

_____ Advance notice required.

PASSION SEEKERS' COUPON ♥

This coupon entitles you to one *photography session* with yours truly as the model.

_____ Advance notice required.

PASSION SEEKERS' COUPONS TO GIVE TO HER

PASSION SEEKERS' COUPON ♥
This coupon entitles you to one *romantic and passionate date* with your mate, entirely planned and orchestrated by yours truly.
_____ Advance notice required.

PASSION SEEKERS' COUPON ♥
This coupon entitles you to receive from me a *massage and oil rubdown* with no strings attached.
_____ Advance notice required.

♥
PASSION SEEKERS' COUPON
This coupon entitles you to a *bedroom story* narrated by yours truly.
No advance notice required.

♥
PASSION SEEKERS' COUPON
This coupon entitles you to ___ minutes of *oral sex.*
No advance notice required.

♥
PASSION SEEKERS' COUPON
This coupon entitles you to ___ minutes of *extended foreplay.*
No advance notice required.

PASSION SEEKERS' COUPON ♥
Master, this coupon entitles you to *one half hour of slavery* by yours truly.
No advance notice required.

♥
PASSION SEEKERS' COUPON
Master, this coupon entitles you to *one hour of slavery* by yours truly.
_____ Advance notice required.

♥
PASSION SEEKERS' COUPON
This coupon entitles you to _____ with yours truly.
_____ Advance notice required.